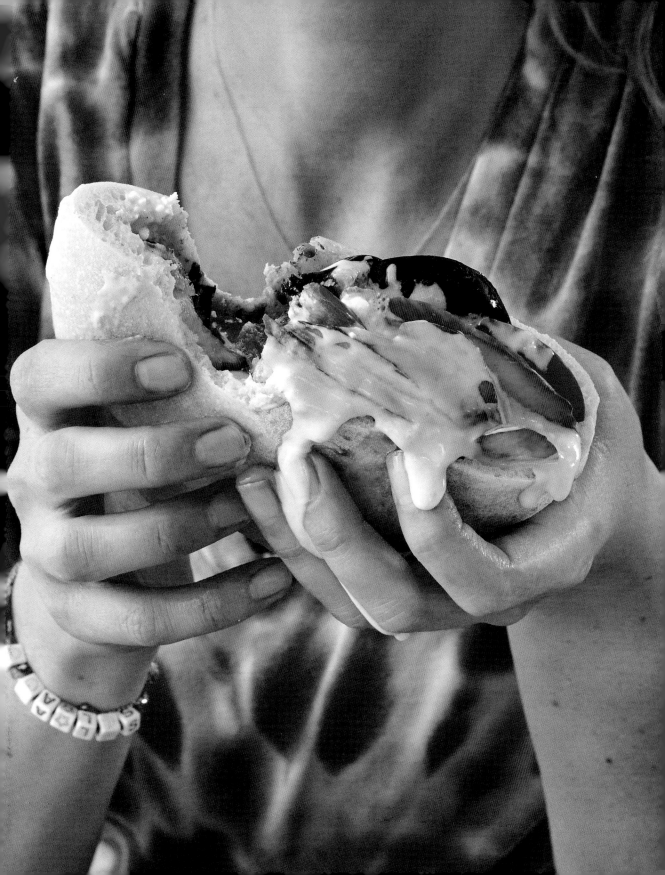

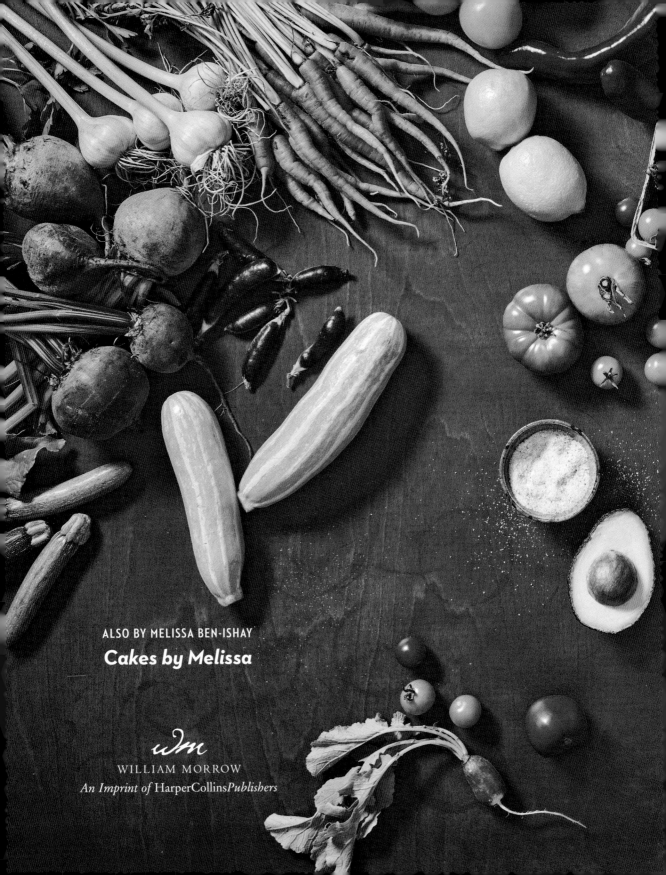

ALSO BY MELISSA BEN-ISHAY

Cakes by Melissa

WM
WILLIAM MORROW
An Imprint of HarperCollinsPublishers

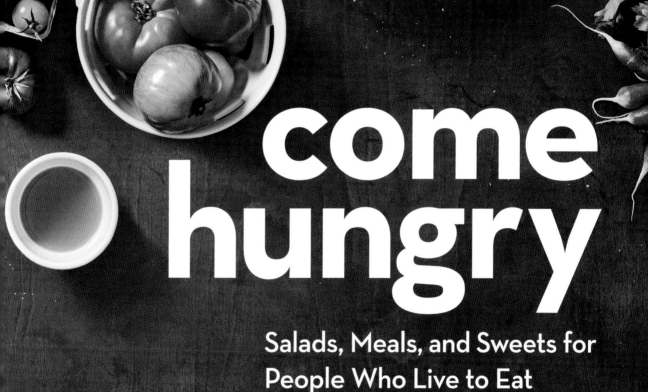

come hungry

Salads, Meals, and Sweets for
People Who Live to Eat

Melissa Ben-Ishay

Photography by Ashley Sears

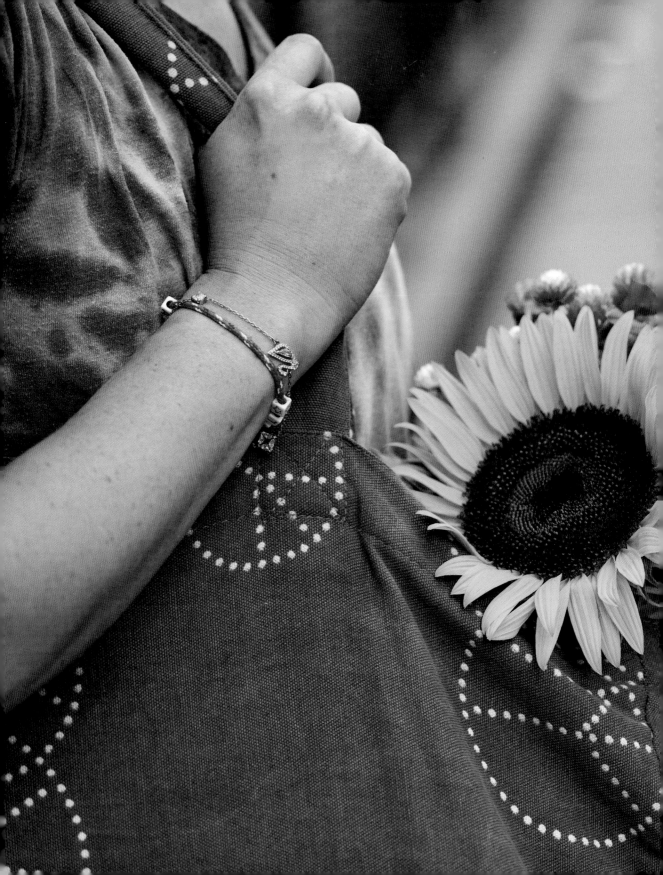

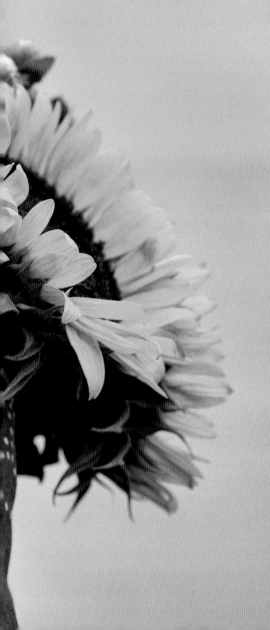

For Adi, this is our book.
Thank you for being my muse.

For Lennie & Scottie:
Eat the rainbow.

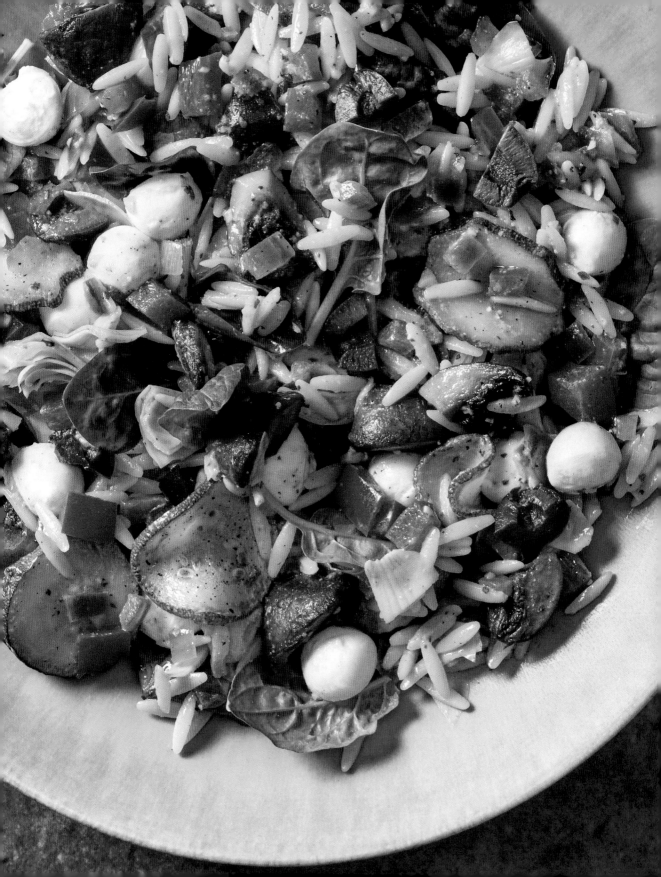

contents

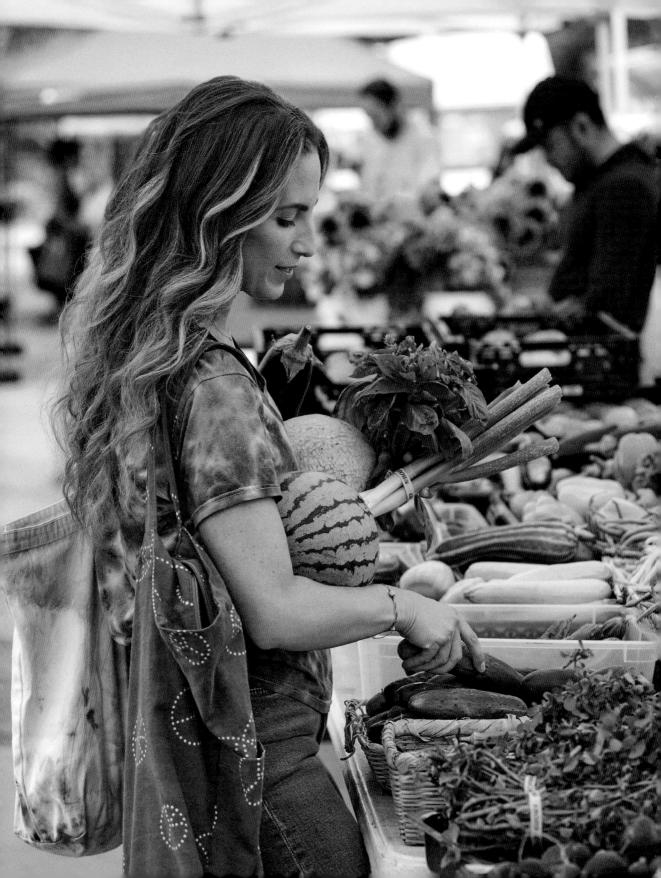

introduction

my food philosophy Mealtime is for nourishment and dessert is for indulging. If you get your nourishment from mealtime, you can absolutely indulge in dessert every day, just like I do.

Two garlic cloves, one small shallot, the juice of two lemons, chives, ¼ cup olive oil, splash of rice vinegar, walnuts, cashews, basil and spinach, nutritional yeast, salt to taste . . . that is so good.

You could call it the salad that started a movement. One night, my husband, Adi, and I were going next door to have a pizza party in our friend's backyard, and I decided to use what I had in the fridge to make a salad. I chopped the green cabbage, cucumbers, and scallions super fine and based the creamy, bright green dressing on my tried-and-true vegan pesto recipe. By the time it was assembled, it almost looked more like a dip than a salad. I took one bite and exclaimed, "Oh my God!"—it was just that good. My friends and I finished the whole bowl in one sitting, some of us eating it with tortilla chips and others serving heaping spoonfuls of it as a side salad. Every now and then you make something on a whim that turns out to be mind-blowingly delicious, and that night, we all knew that this was a *hit*.

Because we all loved that Green Goddess salad so much, I kept making it, and soon after, I posted a video with the recipe on TikTok. I never could've anticipated the response—that one video now has 25 million views, landed me on the *Today* show, was featured on *Live with Kelly and Ryan*, and swept social media with other creators making their own version, even Lizzo and Cardi B. It was so cool and totally unexpected.

In a lot of ways, the Green Goddess gave me permission to write this cookbook filled with the savory recipes I love so much that I make them every day. It's truly a dream come true.

here's to you, green goddess. thank you for everything.

With a dressing packed with greens and bursting with bright flavors, the Green Goddess is the perfect embodiment of my food philosophy: mealtime is for nourishment and dessert is for indulging. If you get your nourishment from mealtime, you can absolutely indulge in dessert every day, just like I do.

The recipes I've included in this book are delicious and they make you feel great. They're packed with flavor, are fast to make, and allow vibrant, nourishing produce to shine. I've always loved to cook, but my approach to food truly transformed when I met

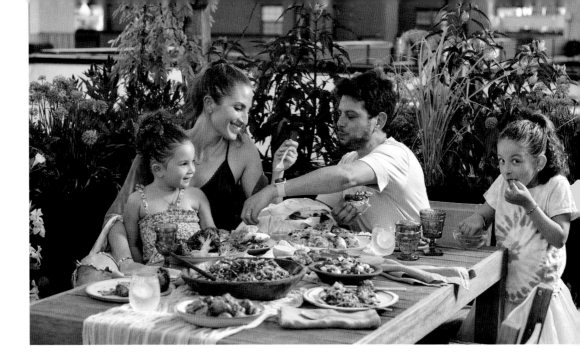

Adi and his mother, Ruthie, who are from Israel. They taught me a different style of cooking—and with it, a whole new way to eat. They start each meal with a spread of colorful, satisfying small plates filled with a variety of spices and flavors, like the Roasted Red Pepper Salad (page 26) and Eggplant Dip (page 29), saving the extras to eat throughout the week in pitas or on toast.

My everyday cooking is absolutely inspired by everyone who has ever invited me into the kitchen with them, including my parents, grandparents, husband, and in-laws. From my grandmother's bungalow colony in the Catskills to my in-laws' home on the Mediterranean, I learned about flavor combinations that excite your taste buds, techniques that make cooking easy, and the generosity that invites everyone to "**come hungry**." All are equally important in a nourishing kitchen and have helped me grow into the cook I am today.

When I was growing up in New Jersey, I helped my mom make dinner every night. She'd pull a chair up to the counter so I could help her make dessert while she whisked together balsamic vinaigrette with a packet of seasoning. (Remember those?) The recipes she cooked for us day in and out inspired the Crunchy Ramen Slaw with Grilled Ribeye (page 65) and the Green Goddess Pasta Salad (page 164), along with countless others.

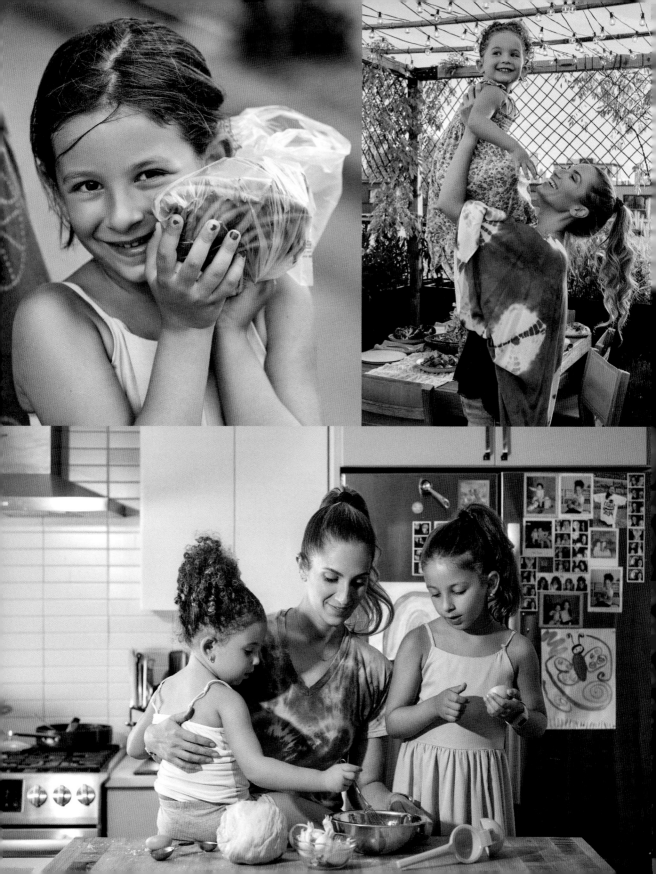

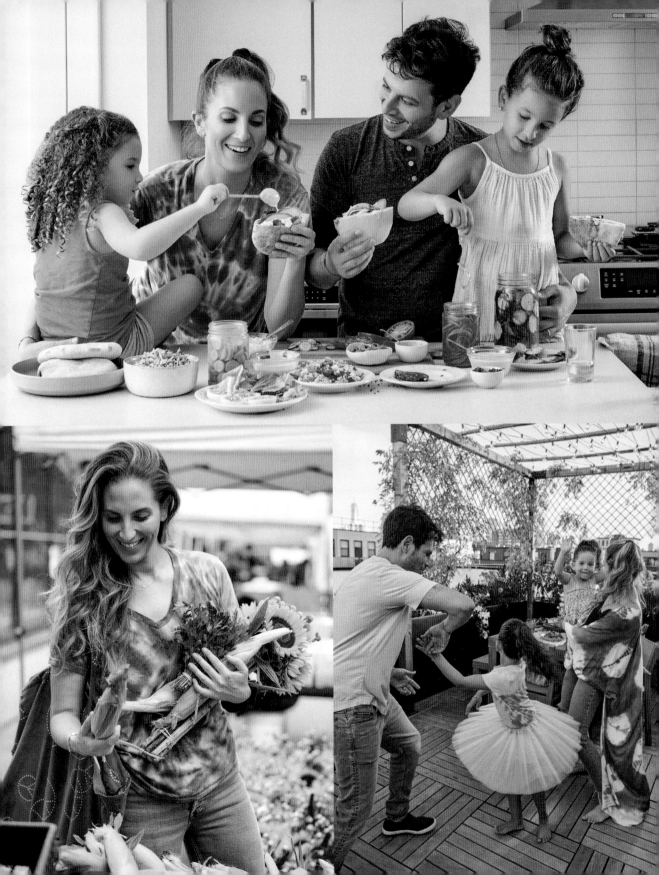

While my mom spent hours in the kitchen patiently teaching me, I inherited my love for food from my dad. He famously tells us stories about how, as a child (and the youngest of four boys), he would sit down at the table and ask, "If I want more, can I have more?" before he took his first bite of any meal. He's still the first one to finish his meals, crediting his quick eating to being the youngest in the family.

Both of my grandmothers were born in Brooklyn and raised their families in Queens. Their children—my aunt and uncles, mom and dad—all have strong Queens accents, and if I close my eyes, I can hear their voices vividly. Soda was "soder," pizza was "pizzer." If you're on your way over, the first thing any of us will tell you to bring either in an accent or not, spoken or implied—is nothing: "Just **come hungry**." We all insist our guests arrive with an appetite, and we mean it.

The women in my family are *balaboostas*. The old-school definition of the Yiddish term means "perfect homemaker," but I much prefer a more modern spin—a woman who appears to effortlessly lead a household and career while nourishing loved ones with delicious, vibrant recipes (it's definitely not effortless). I, too, am a balaboosta.

Growing up, I spent summers visiting my maternal grandparents at their bungalow in the Catskills. My grandma Sylvia (my mom's mom) always enlisted my help making salads filled with roughly chopped iceberg and big chunks of cucumbers. I'd eagerly dip the greens in ranch or creamy Italian dressing to snack on as I cut. The kitchen was tiny—the counter wasn't much wider than the salad bowl I stood over—so I still can't get over the fact that she relinquished control of the salad to a four-year-old standing on a chair. Now, I think she must've seen something in me even then—she must've known I'd grow up to find therapy in the rhythmic sounds of the knife swinging against a cutting board. I was a balaboosta in training.

My dad's mom, my grandma Annie, could be home at 5 p.m. and have a five-course meal on the table by 6:30. And she made it look effortless. Many of the family recipes that have been passed down over the years come from her kitchen. Annie made delicious meals for a crowd with ease, from her famous chocolate cake (which I included in my first cookbook, *Cakes by Melissa*) to chopped liver and brisket at large holiday meals. She thrived on chaos, raising four sons in a small house in Queens. I remember running around her kitchen with my brother and cousins while she cooked, unfazed. She's my inspiration.

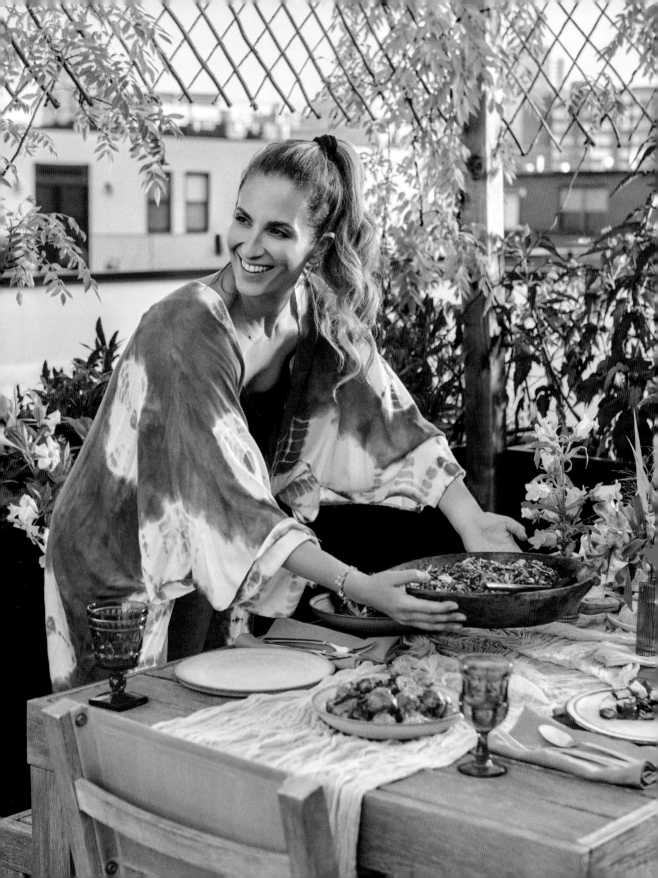

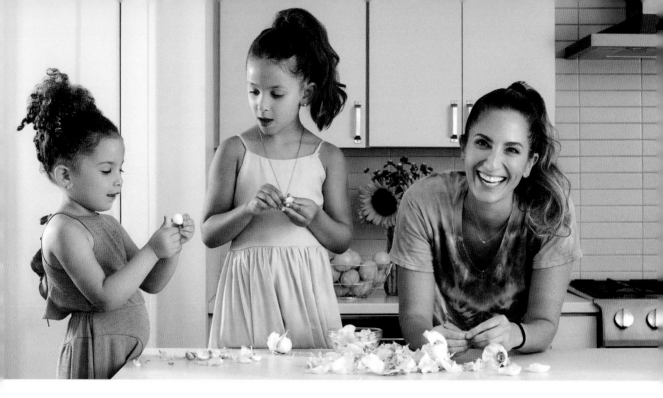

I often think of my grandma Annie in the chaos of my own kitchen as I make dinner for Adi and our daughters. As a mother of two girls, I know how much patience it takes to cook with kids, which makes me even more grateful that my parents and grandparents spent time empowering me in the kitchen. Now, my oldest daughter, Scottie, comes running when she hears the jingle of chocolate chips in a jar; and my youngest, Lennie, eagerly cracks any egg open for me. She's gotten pretty good at it.

All the same, my daughters still don't eat all the recipes in this book. I hope that through leading by example and instilling in them a love of fresh, delicious food, someday they will. I tell them daily that they can do anything, and with any luck, that will include eating their greens while they rule the world.

Adi and I have a shared passion for food. He loves breakfast, I love dinner. We are opposites in so many ways, but happily, opposites attract. When we first started dating, we'd spend hours in the kitchen making dinner for our friends and family. His Mediterranean approach to cooking is what pivoted mine into a healthier direction, with techniques like using extra virgin olive oil instead of butter and adding lemon juice to brighten flavors. The dishes we make are delicious *and* nourishing. Everyone keeps eating them because they taste so good, not just because they're good for you.

In our first apartment in Manhattan's Chelsea neighborhood, we would regularly host loud, joyful, delicious meals. This was before we had kids, which meant our whole day could be spent cutting up vegetables for the Mediterranean Chopped Salad (page 97) or marinating the ingredients for the Grilled Veggies & Halloumi (page 150). Every time someone asked us what they could bring, it was always the same. "Nothing, just come hungry." And then I'd chuckle, thinking of my mom, aunt, and grandmas all saying the same exact thing.

Everyone who knows me knows I measure more with my heart than with a tablespoon. If you're comfortable in the kitchen, I encourage you to do the same, especially when it comes to garlic. Explore new colors and new produce. Go to the market and see what inspires you. Cook outside of your comfort zone. And devour the recipes in this book (which obviously contain measurements)—they'll introduce you to new dishes and new ways of cooking with vegetables while you eat really freaking delicious meals.

This book is filled with more than recipes: It shares a way of eating that prioritizes nourishing ingredients in every meal. I always keep a few of the dishes from the Small Plates section in my fridge for a quick lunch or to make the toasts you'll find in the Toasts section. I wake up every day thinking about what I'll have for lunch, and many of the salads and sides—filled with hearty grains, flavorful proteins, and colorful produce—end up on the menu, especially if I'm feeding a group. And we hardly ever sit down for dinner without bread, so Adi shared many of his "famous" bread recipes with me to share with you.

For dessert, I can't resist a creamy Cookies & Cream Icebox Cake (page 217) or gooey Cookie Butter Blondies (page 229). I'm a dessert person to my bones, and these recipes include a few tricks I use to create more healthy treats that still satisfy my sweet tooth.

Finally, if you're as brave as my mom and grandma Sylvia and want to welcome your little ones into the kitchen, my tips for eliciting their help can be found in the Kitchen Basics section toward the end (see page 253).

Get ready to discover new favorite recipes that nourish you—body *and* soul. I hope you're hungry.

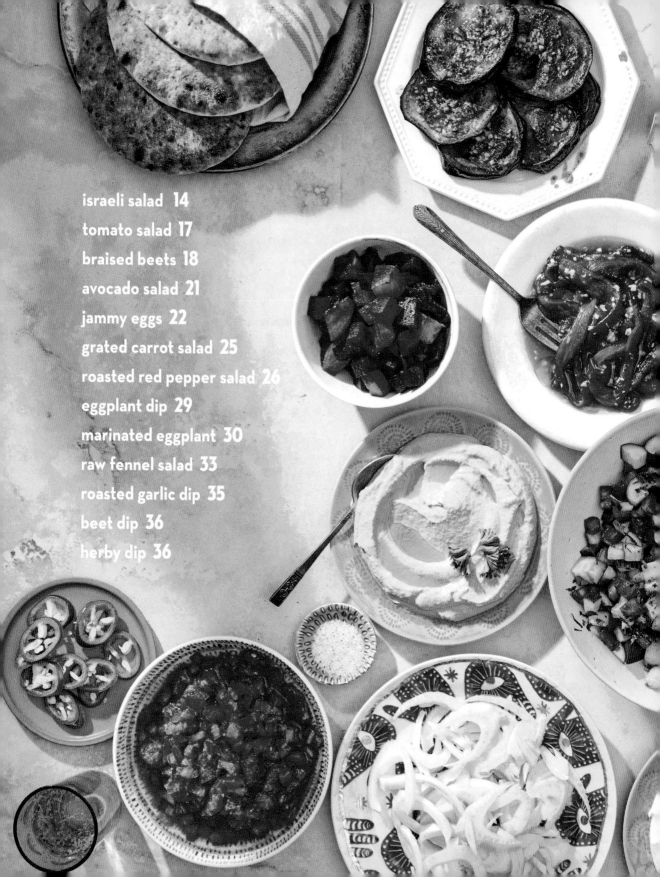

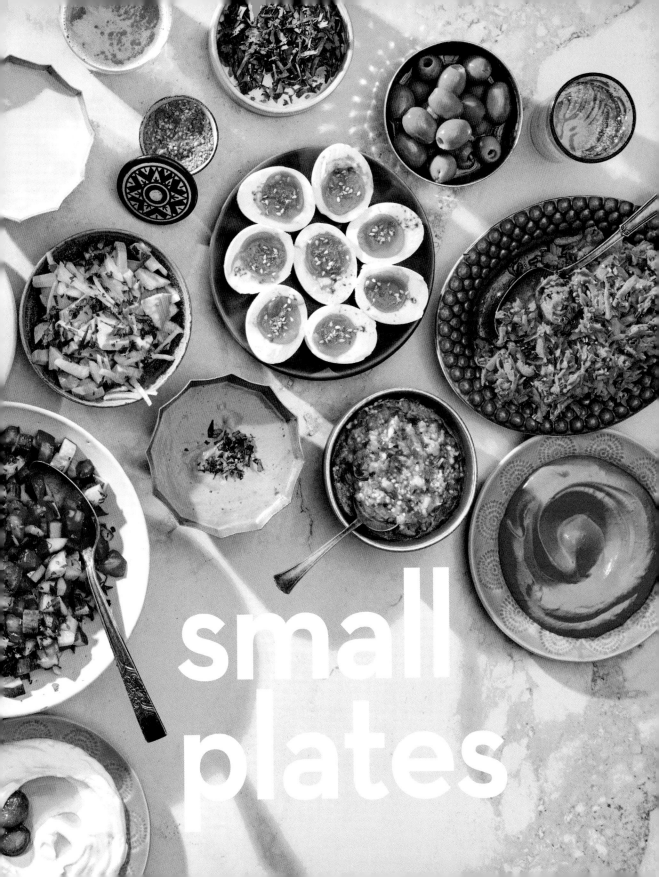

small
plates

Adi took me to visit his family in Israel for the first time for Passover in 2010, when we had been dating for about a year. His mom greeted us with one of the most beautiful spreads I had ever seen. The table was brimming with small bowls filled with mouthwatering salads and dips. A pile of freshly made pita sat on the side, waiting to be torn into and filled with everything on the table. It was love at first sight (and it's maybe even the reason I married my husband).

My in-laws live in a charming apartment just a few minutes away from the Mediterranean. It's on the ground level with a big backyard, and the place always smells like whatever my mother-in-law is cooking. But it's the delicious ingredients and the love that Adi's parents show through food that make it feel like home. I swear, the produce in Israel just tastes better—the tomatoes burst with sugary juices, cucumbers aren't watery, and red peppers have a citrusy sweetness. The vegetables are so delicious I dream about them whenever we aren't there, which is too often.

Israel's cuisine is undoubtedly influenced by neighboring Middle Eastern countries. Regional variations can determine what herbs are used, the preparation methods, and what's served on the side. No two eggplant dips are the same because most people use recipes passed down by their moms or grandmothers. I think it's beautiful to see so many different cultures embracing the same ingredients and recipes as their ancestors to create truly delicious meals. That's exactly what you'll find in this section—family recipes inspired by life in Israel and by Jewish heritage.

My favorite part of visiting my in-laws is Shabbat dinner. My mother-in-law spends all day Friday chopping, dicing, and roasting vegetables in preparation for friends and family to join; everyone who comes brings something different. The weather is always beautiful, so we eat outside in the backyard at a long table, with each small plate appearing in no fewer than three separate bowls so everyone can reach them easily from where they are sitting. On top of the dozens of small bowls scattered around the table, there's a large dish in the middle of the table with enough for everyone to share. If generosity weren't the theme of this weekly gathering, variety would be. My mother-in-law and I share the same love language—cooking for others—so even when I'm stuffed with vegetables by the time the main course rolls around, I make room for the entire meal so I can appreciate every bite.

Visiting Israel transformed how I nourish myself. Now, indulging in a colorful variety of small plates is without a doubt one of my favorite ways to eat. As a result, I eat a vegetable-heavy diet that makes me feel fulfilled and like I'm wasting less because whatever isn't eaten at dinner gets saved in the fridge for grazing throughout the week, to be used as a condiment or to snack on. All the recipes work for breakfast, lunch, or dinner—they're delicious on their own, stuffed into a pita, or to zhuzh up a salad. Sometimes, breakfast means a pita filled with Israeli salad, marinated eggplant, and tahina. Other times, it's a bowl of cottage cheese with braised beets. But my number one rule? Eat what's delicious and makes you feel good.

❝Indulging in a colorful variety of small plates is without a doubt one of my favorite ways to eat. ❞

israeli salad

I could drink this salad like water. You may also know it as a Shirazi, Persian, or Arabic salad, but I grew up calling it an Israeli salad (though the names are different, the ingredients are mostly the same). Every time we come back from visiting Adi's family, I want to eat this salad every day. There's so much to love about it, from the finely chopped vegetables to the simple dressing. The first time I had an Israeli salad was a big aha moment for me because I realized that when you use the highest-quality produce, you need only extra virgin olive oil, lemon, and salt to highlight the ingredients and show you the power of Mother Nature. **SERVES 4 TO 6**

4 Roma tomatoes (or 2 large farm stand tomatoes, in season), finely chopped

½ red onion, finely chopped

6 Persian cucumbers, finely chopped

Juice of 1 lemon (about 3 tablespoons)

2 tablespoons chopped fresh parsley

3 tablespoons extra virgin olive oil

½ teaspoon fine sea salt

1. In a large bowl, combine the tomatoes, red onion, and cucumbers.

2. In a small bowl, whisk together the lemon juice, parsley, olive oil, and salt.

3. Pour the dressing over the vegetables and gently stir to combine.

4. Season to taste and serve immediately. Store any leftover salad in the fridge in an airtight container for 3 to 5 days.

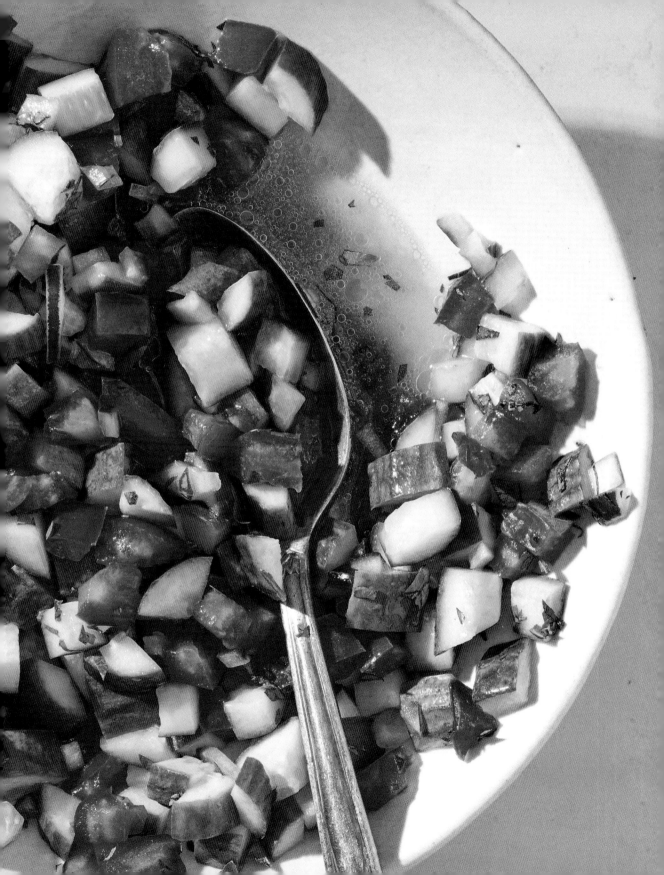

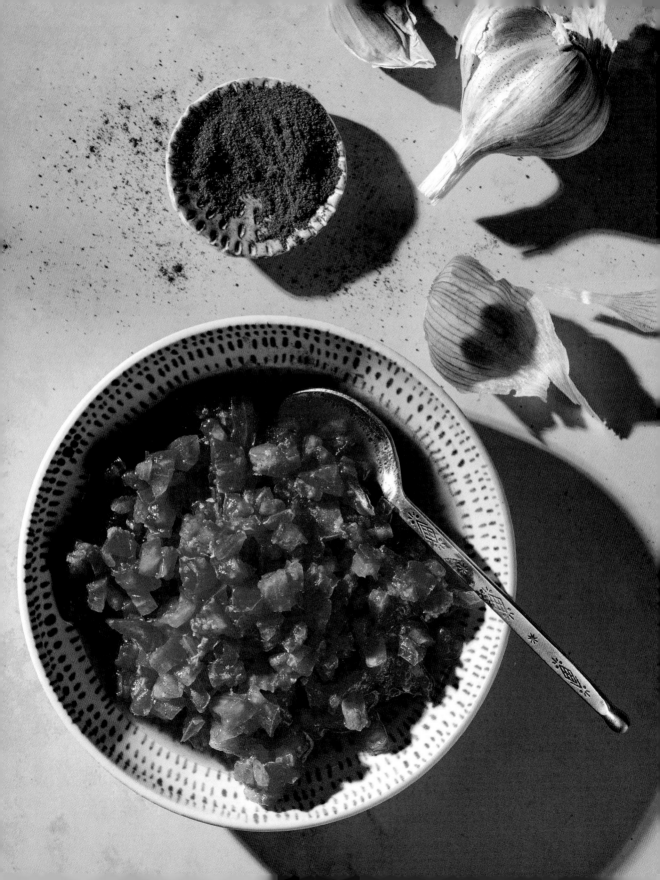

tomato salad

I normally take out the tomato seeds when making this salad, but if you like them, keep them in. However you make it, I'd recommend doubling the recipe, so you can use the leftovers as a condiment for sandwiches all week long. When I make it, I always use sweet paprika with oil—the added oil gives it a burst of flavor and aroma you don't get with regular paprika. This salad is simple, delicious, and holds a special place in my heart because Adi made it all the time when we first started dating.

SERVES 4 TO 6

4 Roma tomatoes (or 2 large farm stand tomatoes, in season), finely chopped

1 teaspoon fine sea salt

Juice of 1 lemon (about 3 tablespoons)

1 tablespoon extra virgin olive oil

2 garlic cloves, grated with a Microplane

1 tablespoon sweet paprika with oil

Combine the tomatoes, salt, lemon juice, oil, garlic, and paprika in a large bowl and toss gently. Season to taste and serve immediately. Store any leftovers in an airtight container in the fridge for 3 to 5 days.

tip: Use leftovers to make the Avocado & Tomato Toast (page 48).

braised beets

Beets are naturally sweet and a touch earthy, and the onion in this recipe adds a great depth of flavor. I often make this salad when I'm not feeling my best because it creates a comforting, nourishing meal without making me feel too full. My secret is to eat it on top of a big dollop of cottage cheese for a light but satisfying meal. **SERVES 4 TO 6**

4 large beets, peeled

3 tablespoons extra virgin olive oil

1 large red onion, roughly chopped

1 teaspoon fine sea salt

¼ teaspoon freshly ground black pepper

1½ cups vegetable broth

Cottage cheese, for serving (optional)

1. Cut the beets into ½-inch discs, then into matchsticks ½ inch wide.

2. Heat the olive oil in a large skillet over medium heat. Add the onion and sauté until translucent, about 8 minutes. Season with the salt and pepper.

3. Add the beets and cook for 3 to 5 minutes to fully coat them with the onion and oil, stirring occasionally so they don't burn. Pour in the vegetable broth and cover.

4. Bring the liquid to a boil, then lower the heat to medium to low and cook until the beets are tender, about 35 minutes. Uncover the pan and cook until the liquid has reduced by half, about 10 minutes more.

5. Season to taste and serve the beets immediately as a side or over cottage cheese. Store any leftovers in the fridge in an airtight container for 3 to 5 days and use to top salads and sandwiches.

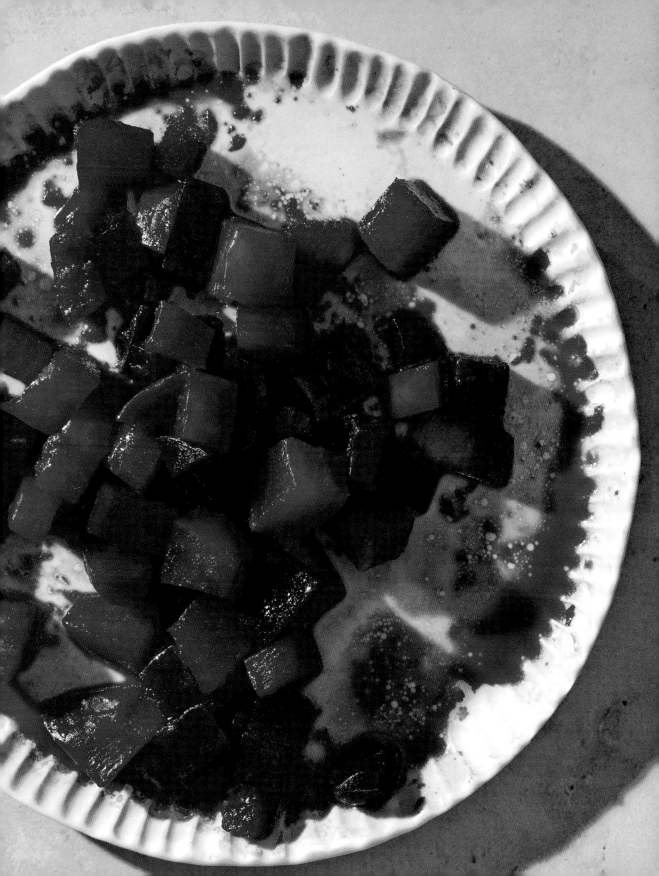

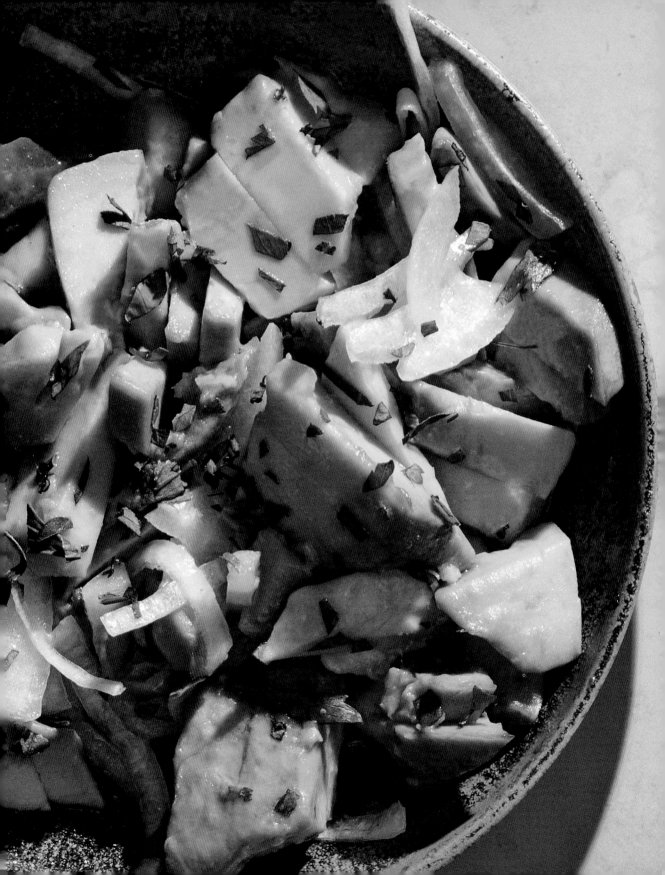

avocado salad

You could, of course, call this salad guacamole (especially since I've been known to eat it with a chip), but I classify it as a salad because of the way I assemble it. You can prepare the dressing in advance but wait to dice the avocado and onion until just before you're ready to serve to keep the avocado nice and bright. No matter what you call it, it makes a great meal on its own or to garnish another salad, especially the Vegan Taco Salad on page 77. **SERVES 4 TO 6**

Juice of 2 lemons (about ⅓ cup)

2 tablespoons extra virgin olive oil

1 tablespoon chopped fresh parsley

1 tablespoon chopped fresh cilantro

½ teaspoon fine sea salt

¼ teaspoon freshly ground black pepper

2 ripe avocados

½ white onion

1. Whisk together the lemon juice, olive oil, herbs, salt, and pepper in a small bowl.

2. Just before serving, halve and pit the avocados. Carefully score each side of the avocado, first vertically, then horizontally, to create ¼-inch to ½-inch cubes. Scoop the avocado into a medium bowl with a large spoon.

3. Dice the onion into ¼-inch to ½-inch pieces (to match the avocado) and add to the bowl. Combine gently (you want the avocado to keep its shape, not get mashed).

4. Stir in the dressing and serve immediately.

jammy eggs

When you eat a vegetable-forward diet, by default people always ask where you get your protein. Of course, there are so many different ways to add protein to salads, but I'll rarely add an ingredient that doesn't elevate the dish in some way or enhance the overall taste. Cue jammy eggs. Classic Israeli breakfasts (as I've experienced them) always feature eggs in some way, whether in an omelet, over easy, or jammy. I make mine the way Adi grew up eating them: sprinkled with a pinch of sesame seeds, sea salt, and cumin. It's one of the recipes in this chapter that's extra special to our home, like the dips, which makes me love it even more. Use these eggs for the Kale Cobb Salad with Crispy Shallots (page 80) or add them to a pita filled with vegetables for a fast, filling weekend lunch. I find brown eggs far easier to peel than white eggs, so I always make sure to get those when I plan to boil them. **MAKES 6 EGGS**

6 large brown eggs

1. Bring a large pot of water to a rolling boil. Carefully add the eggs with a slotted spoon and cook for 7 minutes.

2. Meanwhile, prepare an ice bath in a large bowl.

3. Remove the eggs from the boiling water and immediately transfer them to the ice bath. Let the eggs cool for at least 1 minute to make them easier to peel. If not eating immediately, refrigerate the eggs in the shells for up to 1 week.

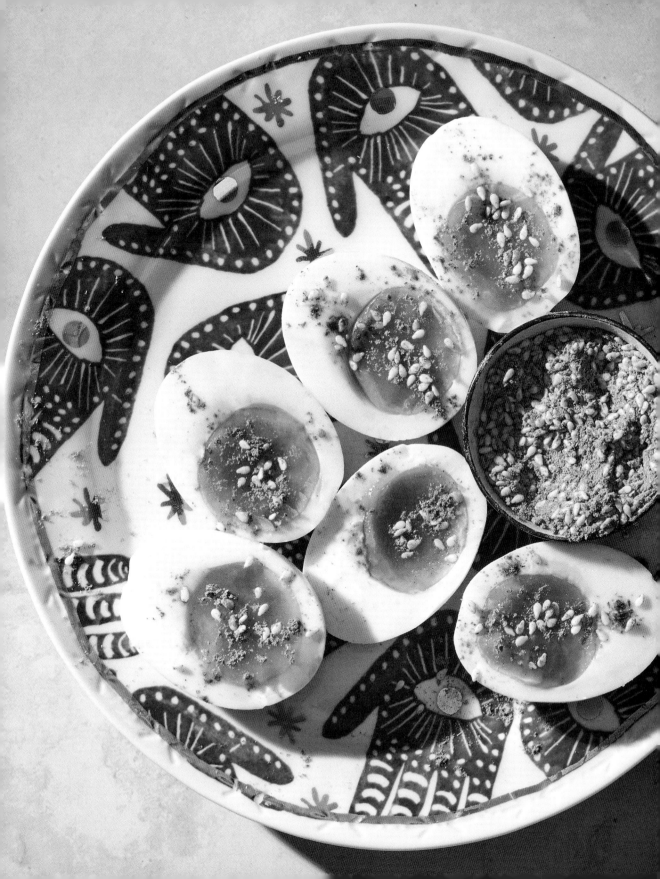

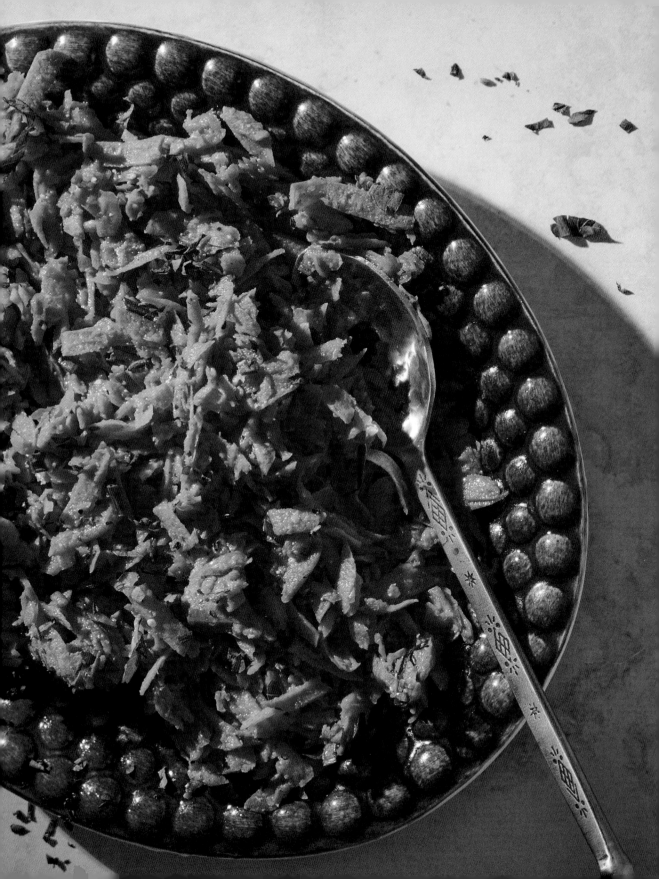

grated carrot salad

Carrots are the only vegetable loved (or at least liked) by everyone in my house. The ones I order from Lancaster Farms, a sustainable farming co-op in Pennsylvania, are the best, most delicious ones I've ever had, so I add them to my cart at least once a week. This salad is great on its own, or it can be added to wraps, salads, or sandwiches. If you can find fresh, locally grown carrots for this recipe, please use them, because it will make the salad infinitely more flavorful. I prefer to use stone-ground German mustard for its added hint of spice, but you can use Dijon, too. Grated carrot salads are also an ideal side for a protein-heavy meal, like grilled fish or chicken, or even as a simple pita filling. **SERVES 4 TO 6**

8 medium carrots, peeled

1½ tablespoons chopped fresh parsley, plus more for garnish

1½ tablespoons chopped fresh chives, plus more for garnish

FOR THE DRESSING

3 tablespoons extra virgin olive oil

1 tablespoon German mustard

1 teaspoon honey

Juice of 1 lemon (about 3 tablespoons)

½ teaspoon ground cumin

¾ teaspoon fine sea salt

¼ teaspoon freshly ground black pepper

1. Grate the carrots in a food processor or on the larger holes of a box grater. Combine them in a large bowl with the parsley and chives.

2. MAKE THE DRESSING: In a small bowl, whisk together the olive oil, mustard, honey, lemon juice, cumin, salt, and pepper. Add the dressing to the salad and stir to combine.

3. Garnish with parsley and chives and serve. Store any leftovers in a sealed container in the fridge for up to 1 week.

roasted red pepper salad

Adi and I have been making this salad ever since we started living together, but the recipe was taken directly from his mother's kitchen. Once the peppers are roasted, Adi's mother puts them in a grocery store plastic bag to cool—the steam makes the charred skin practically fall off. Another way to achieve the same effect (and my method of choice) is to use a closed glass food storage container. As you slice the roasted peppers, save as much of the juice that spills out as you can—it adds so much flavor to the final dish. **SERVES 4 TO 6**

3 red bell peppers

8 garlic cloves, finely chopped

Juice of 1 lemon (about 3 tablespoons)

1 tablespoon white vinegar

1 tablespoon extra virgin olive oil

1 teaspoon fine sea salt

¼ teaspoon freshly ground black pepper

1. Preheat the oven to broil and place the whole bell peppers on a baking sheet.

2. Broil on high until the outsides are mostly charred. Carefully turn the peppers with tongs to get an even char on all sides.

3. Remove the charred peppers from the oven and carefully place in a sealed container to cool (this makes them easier to peel).

4. Once you can safely handle the peppers, peel off the charred outside with your fingers. It should come off easily. Keep as much of the juice from the peppers as you can.

5. Slice the peppers into thin strips, discarding the centers. In a large bowl, combine the pepper slices and chopped garlic.

6. Add the lemon juice, vinegar, olive oil, salt, and pepper, and stir to combine. Adjust seasonings to taste. Store leftovers in an airtight container in the fridge for 3 to 5 days.

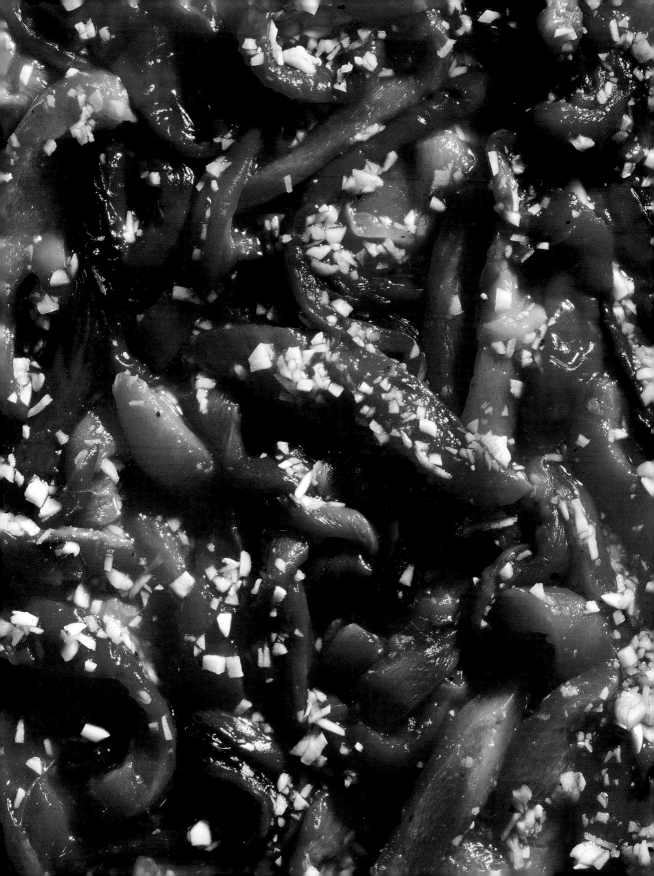

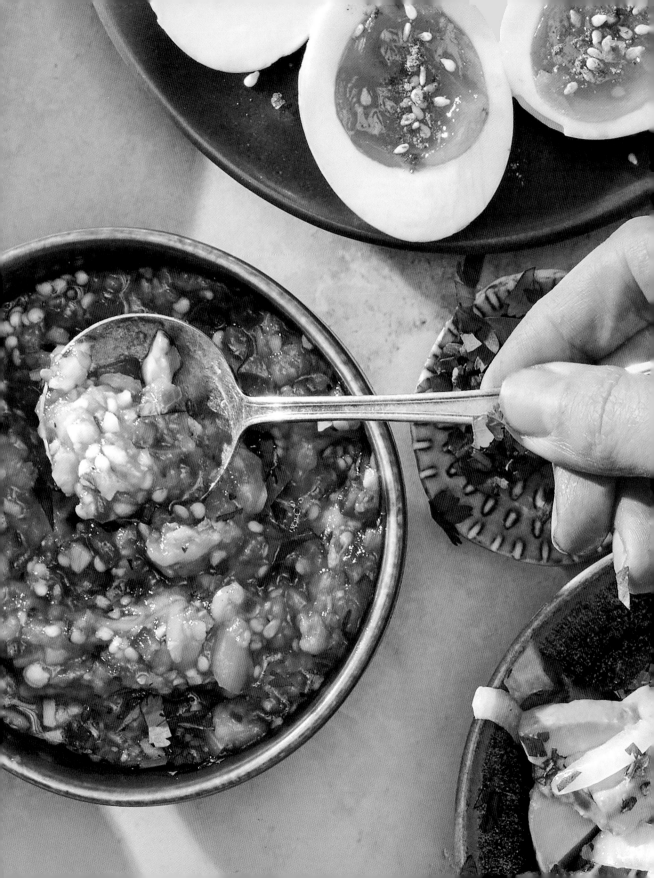

eggplant dip

This dip is inspired by Adi's mom's recipe, with lots of herbs and spices to bring out all of the delicious flavors. I like to make this salad as soon as possible after the eggplant comes out of the oven, so the warmth of the eggplant cooks the garlic and blooms the herby aromas. Enjoy it with a fresh pita, tahina, cucumbers, and the Roasted Red Pepper Salad (page 26). **SERVES 4 TO 6**

1 large eggplant

7 garlic cloves

½ red bell pepper

¼ to ½ jalapeño pepper, seeds removed

3 tablespoons finely chopped fresh parsley

2 tablespoons extra virgin olive oil

Juice of 1 lemon (about 3 tablespoons)

Splash of rice vinegar

1 teaspoon fine sea salt

¼ teaspoon freshly ground black pepper

1. Preheat the oven to 425°F.

2. Wrap the eggplant in aluminum foil and place on a baking sheet. Bake for 40 to 50 minutes, until totally soft inside.

3. While the eggplant is baking, mince the garlic, bell pepper, and jalapeño as finely as possible (they should all be about the same size). Add to a large bowl with the parsley and stir together.

4. Once the eggplant is finished cooking, carefully unwrap it from the foil. Slice it in half lengthwise, scoop out the insides, and discard the skins. Chop the eggplant into fine pieces; it should totally break up. While it's still warm, add the eggplant to the large bowl with the vegetables.

5. Stir in the olive oil, lemon juice, rice vinegar, salt, and pepper, and serve in a small bowl. Store any leftovers in the fridge in an airtight container for 3 to 5 days.

marinated eggplant

Any recipe that requires a lot of patience is a tough one for me—that's typically how you can tell when the origins of a recipe are from my mother-in-law or husband. But this eggplant is so delicious it's worth the time. The eggplant is first pan-fried until golden, then drizzled with a gorgeous paprika vinaigrette that adds a sharp, garlicky flavor to every bite. **SERVES 4 TO 6**

1 large eggplant

1 teaspoon fine sea salt, plus more as needed

½ cup avocado oil, plus more as needed

FOR THE MARINADE

¼ cup extra virgin olive oil

2 teaspoons sweet paprika with oil

5 garlic cloves, finely chopped

Juice of 1 lemon (about 3 tablespoons)

1 teaspoon white vinegar

½ teaspoon fine sea salt

¼ teaspoon freshly ground black pepper

1. Cut the eggplant into ¼-inch slices and lay them flat on a tea towel.

2. Salt the slices liberally, flip, and repeat. Let sit for 20 minutes to 1 hour to draw out the excess water, then pat the eggplant dry.

3. Heat the avocado oil in a large pan over medium to high heat. You'll know it's ready when you add the end of a wooden spoon to the oil and bubbles form around it.

4. Fry the eggplant slices until brown, 8 to 10 minutes on each side. You may need to add a bit more oil as you go since the eggplant will absorb oil. The bottom of the pan should always be completely covered with oil.

5. Remove the eggplant from the pan and rest the slices on a cooling rack.

6. AS THE EGGPLANT COOLS, MAKE THE MARINADE: Whisk together the olive oil, paprika, garlic, lemon juice, vinegar, salt, and pepper.

7. Once cooled, place the eggplant in a shallow container or on a plate and drizzle with the marinade. Season with salt and pepper to taste.

8. Serve the eggplant immediately or store in an airtight container in the fridge for 3 to 5 days. Make sure to keep all the juices from the marinade with the eggplant, spooning more over it as you serve.

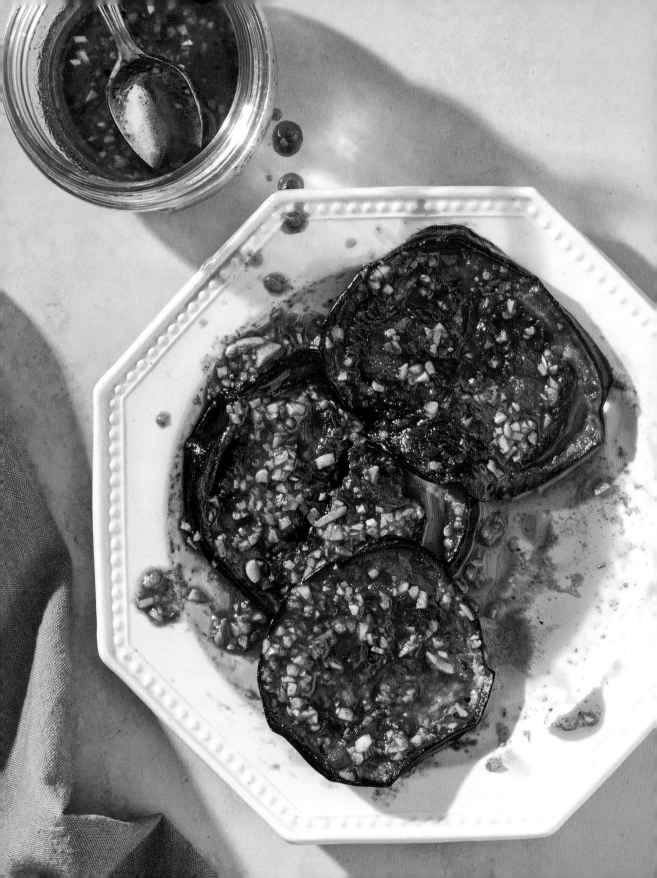

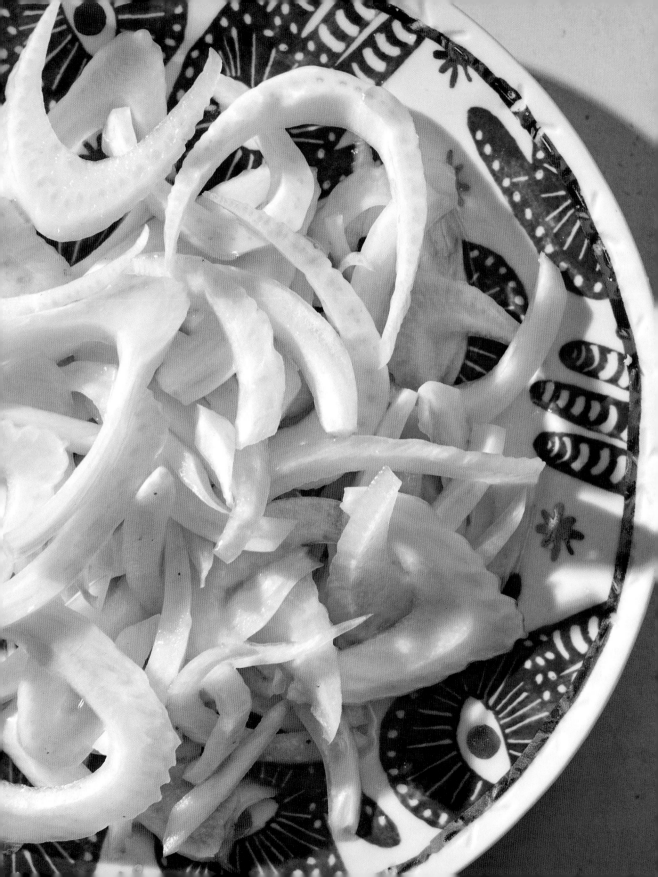

raw fennel salad

Shortly after I became a mom for the first time, Adi did everything he could to feed me things that would increase my milk supply while I was breastfeeding. That's when I started eating fennel—a Mediterranean veggie that's anecdotally known to help produce more breast milk. Honestly, I wouldn't have minded if it were purely anecdotal; this recipe is *that* good. Raw fennel has a crunchy texture and anise-like flavor, so the acid from the lemon juice and peppery extra virgin olive oil here perfectly balance the flavor profile. It may taste complex, but this is truly the easiest thing in the world. Fennel is also high in potassium and fiber, making it even more nourishing, so you can crunch on it all day. **SERVES 4 TO 6**

1 large or 2 small bulbs fennel

Juice of 1 lemon (about 3 tablespoons)

2 tablespoons extra virgin olive oil

½ teaspoon fine sea salt

1. Cut the fronds off the fennel and remove the core. Use a knife or mandoline to cut the fennel into thin slices.

2. Place the fennel in a bowl and cover with the lemon juice, olive oil, and salt. Stir to combine. Serve immediately and store any leftovers in the fridge in an airtight container for 3 to 5 days.

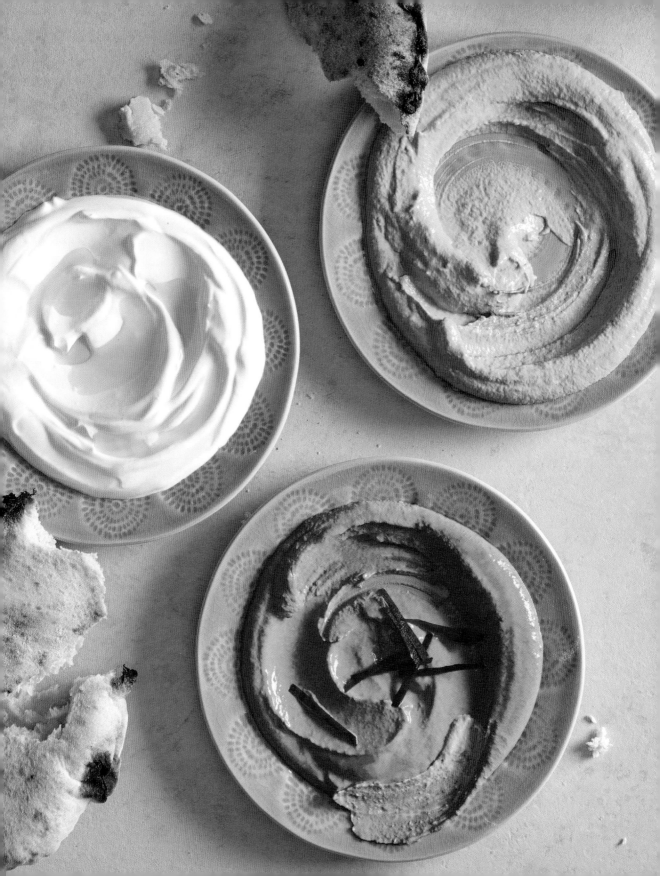

a trio of dips

Knowing how to whip up a delicious dip is one of the best skills a cook can have, and it often doesn't require a lot of ingredients. Many dips start with a creamy base, bright citrus, and an allium (like garlic, caramelized onions, scallions, etc.) for flavor. This trio of beautiful dips all started with one ingredient I always have in my fridge: whole milk cottage cheese. I love cottage cheese and could eat it plain, on toast, or with cucumbers and tomatoes. But blending it was a revelation! Full-fat cottage cheese–based dips are ultra-creamy and packed with protein (low-fat varieties can be more watery), making them perfect for spreading over a sandwich or serving as an appetizer. No matter how I eat it, whole milk cottage cheese from Good Culture is my favorite. If you've never tried cottage cheese, make sure to give it a chance. It's more versatile than people give it credit for. **EACH RECIPE YIELDS 2 CUPS DIP**

roasted garlic dip

2 heads garlic, cloves separated and peeled

½ cup extra virgin olive oil, plus more for garnish

Juice of 1 lemon (about 3 tablespoons)

½ teaspoon fine sea salt

One 16-ounce container whole milk cottage cheese

1. Preheat the oven to 250°F.

2. Place the garlic in a small, oven-safe container and cover with the olive oil. Roast for about 2 hours, until the garlic is golden and soft. Let cool.

3. Add 10 roasted garlic cloves, the lemon juice, salt, and cottage cheese to a food processor and process just until smooth. Don't overdo it, or it will get too runny.

4. Serve in a shallow bowl and garnish with a swirl of fresh olive oil and the remaining roasted garlic cloves. Store any leftovers in the fridge in an airtight container for up to 5 days. Separation is normal; just give it a quick stir before serving.

(continued)

beet dip

Juice of 2 lemons (about ⅓ cup)

1 small roasted beet, cooled and peeled

½ teaspoon fine sea salt

One 16-ounce container whole milk cottage cheese

Extra virgin olive oil

Flaky sea salt

1. Pulse together the lemon juice, roasted beet, and salt in a food processor until smooth.

2. Add the cottage cheese and process again until smooth. Don't overdo it!

3. Serve in a shallow bowl and garnish with a swirl of olive oil and flaky sea salt. Store any leftovers in the fridge in an airtight container for up to 5 days. Separation is normal; just give it a quick stir before serving.

herby dip

Juice of 2 lemons (about ⅓ cup)

2 large garlic cloves

1 bunch fresh parsley, plus more for garnish

1 bunch fresh cilantro, plus more for garnish

One 16-ounce container whole milk cottage cheese

Extra virgin olive oil

1. Blend the lemon juice, garlic, parsley, and cilantro in a food processor until mostly combined.

2. Add the cottage cheese and pulse again to combine. Don't overdo it!

3. Serve in a shallow bowl and garnish with fresh herbs and a swirl of olive oil. Store any leftovers in the fridge in an airtight container for up to 5 days. Separation is normal; just give it a quick stir before serving.

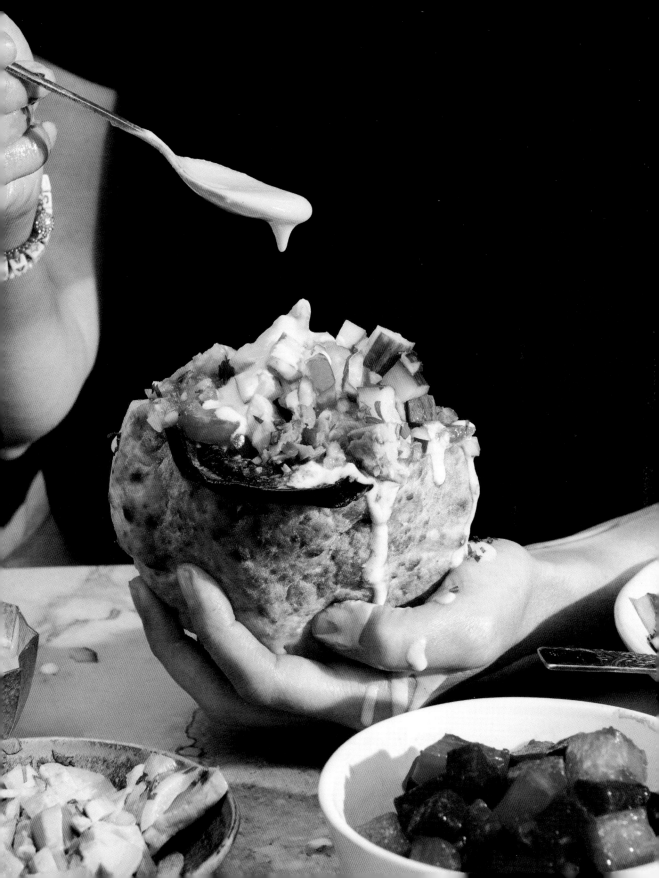

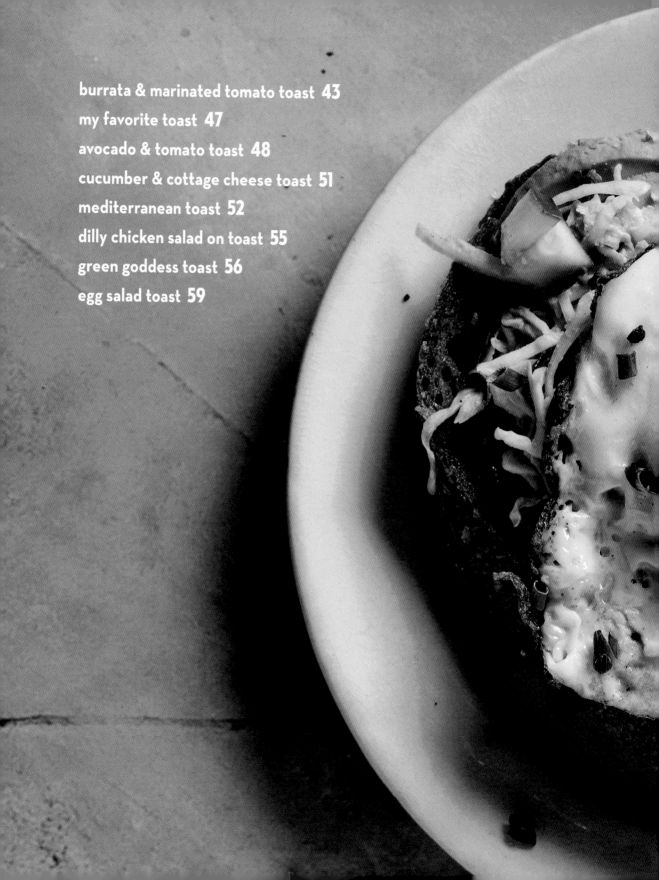

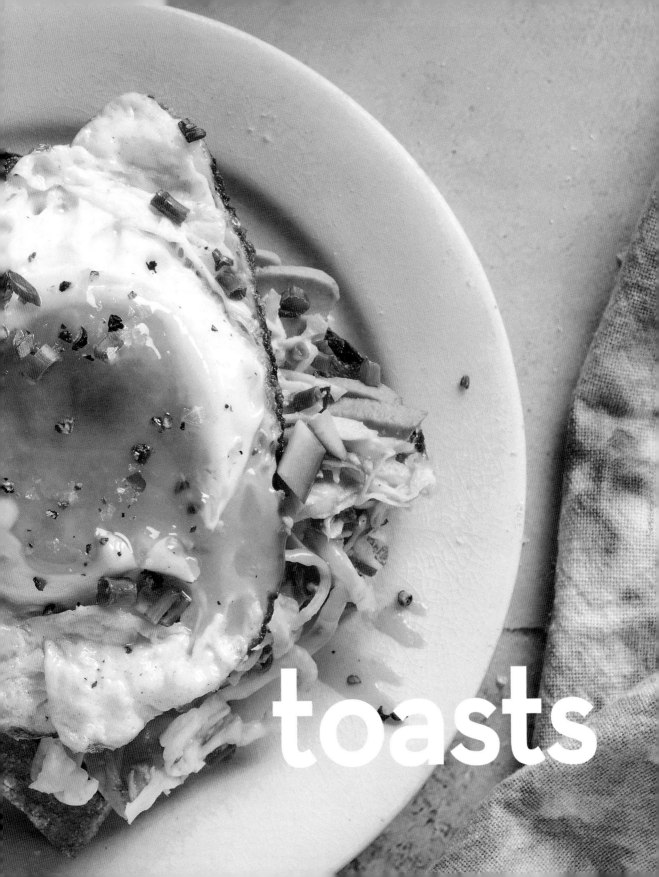

toasts

I wake up each morning thinking about every meal I'm going to eat that day, which shouldn't come as a surprise if you've ever seen me crunch down on a tortilla chip or bite into a golden slice of toast. There's truly no better way to repurpose leftover salad or chopped veggies than by spooning them out onto a freshly toasted piece of sourdough sprinkled with garlic powder or into a fresh pita. I make my own garlic powder (see page 260), which takes time but produces the most flavorful powder in my spice cabinet.

These snacks are designed to help you get the most out of every salad you make. They add flavorful variety to make you excited to open the fridge and see leftovers, especially if you're pressed for time. Don't limit yourself to the combinations listed here—they're a jumping-off point for you to discover your next favorite recipe; any salad you love can be used. One ingredient these recipes share is high-quality extra virgin olive oil. I use Paesanol, a cold-pressed olive oil from Sicily with a rich green color and herbaceous flavor. When buying olive oil, I look for early harvest, cold-pressed oil in an opaque glass bottle—the bottle tells me the elixir is protected from heat and light, which can make it go rancid. A little drizzle of high-quality extra virgin olive oil easily elevates a recipe and creates a flavorful snack with just a few ingredients.

66 These snacks are designed to help you get the most out of every salad you make. 99

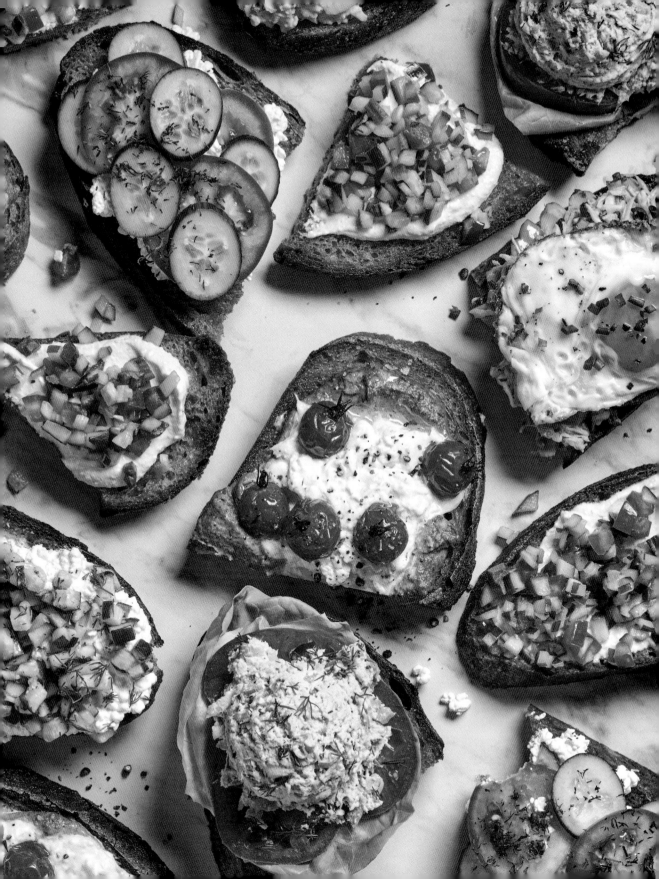

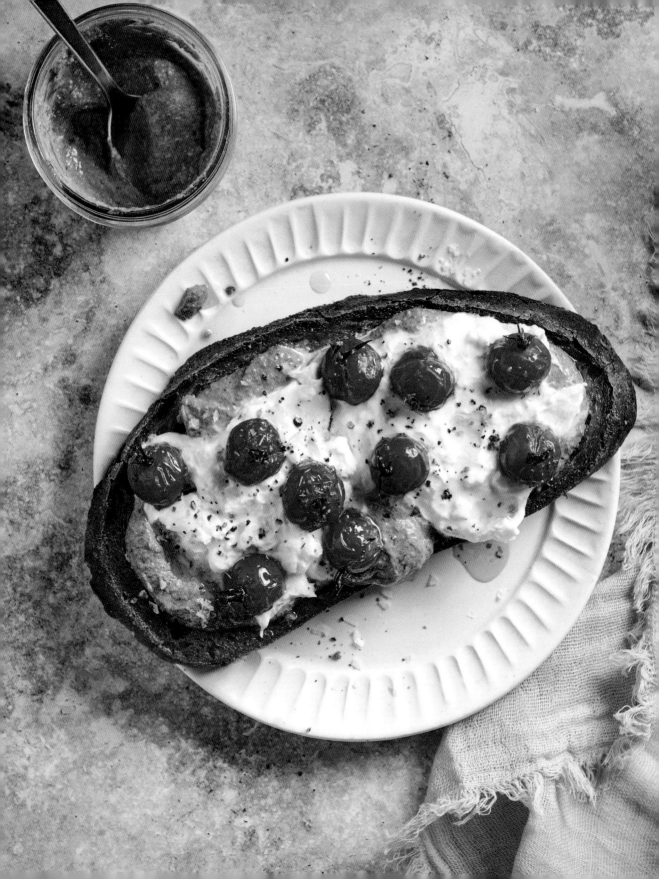

burrata & marinated tomato toast

This recipe is why I started growing fresh basil at home. I always make a double batch of the creamy vegan pesto because, let's face it, it's delicious on just about everything. But making pesto from scratch requires a *lot* of basil, and I always found myself buying the largest quantities possible. If you're able to grow your own basil at home at least part of the year, it will truly transform this recipe—and motivate you to make it more often. Instead of traditional Parmesan, I make it with nutritional yeast, which is one of my favorite ways to add vegan cheesy flavor and extra vitamins to my food. The powdery kitchen staple is gluten- and dairy-free and is packed with B vitamins and amino acids. It's essentially the same yeast used in baking and brewing, but it's fortified and treated to deactivate the yeast. If you don't have any or don't like the taste, it's okay to leave it out.

Pairing the pesto with sweet, acidic cherry tomatoes roasted in olive oil and creamy burrata on crunchy bread creates a next-level appetizer. The small tomatoes swim in extra virgin olive oil, which infuses them with an herbaceous, garlicky flavor as the delicious tomato juices spill out and create a treat for the eyes and taste buds. **SERVES 2**

1 pint cherry tomatoes

4 to 5 garlic cloves

¼ cup extra virgin olive oil

1 teaspoon dried oregano

1 teaspoon fine sea salt

¼ teaspoon freshly ground black pepper

FOR THE CREAMY VEGAN PESTO

2 cups packed fresh basil leaves

Juice of 1½ lemons (about ¼ cup)

3 tablespoons extra virgin olive oil

1 teaspoon fine sea salt

2 garlic cloves

⅓ cup pine nuts

½ cup nutritional yeast

1. Preheat the oven to 400°F.

2. Combine the tomatoes, garlic, olive oil, oregano, salt, and pepper in a baking dish and stir to evenly coat the tomatoes and garlic with seasoning. Bake for 20 to 25 minutes, until the tomatoes and garlic are golden and the tomatoes start to release their juices.

3. MAKE THE PESTO: Add the basil, lemon juice, olive oil, salt, garlic, pine nuts, and nutritional yeast to a food processor or high-powered blender and pulse until smooth. If not using the pesto immediately, store in the fridge in a sealed container for 3 to 5 days.

(continued)

FOR THE TOAST

1 teaspoon extra virgin olive oil, plus more for serving

2 slices fresh sourdough bread

Garlic powder, to taste

One 4-ounce ball fresh burrata

Flaky sea salt

4. NOW, ASSEMBLE THE TOAST: Heat the olive oil in a large skillet over medium-high heat. Pan-fry the bread until golden brown, 4 to 5 minutes per side. Remove the toast from the pan and season with garlic powder.

5. Spread a layer of pesto on the toast.

6. Open the burrata on the toast and spread evenly across. Depending on the size of the burrata, you may only need half.

7. Spoon a few (or more) of the roasted tomatoes and garlic, if desired, on top of the burrata.

8. Sprinkle with flaky sea salt and a drizzle of olive oil to serve. Save any remaining tomatoes in the fridge in an airtight container for 3 to 5 days to eat on toast or with cottage cheese.

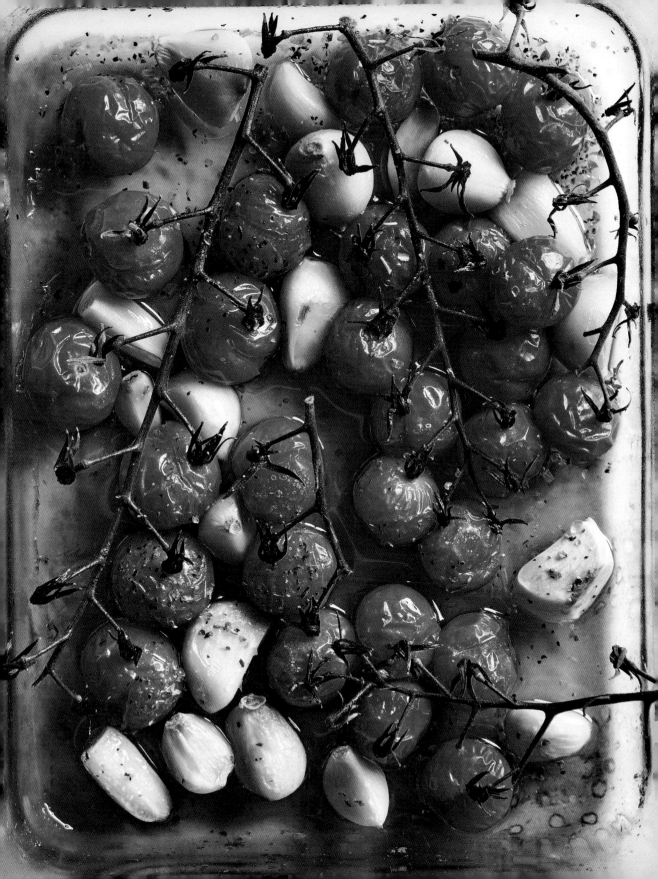

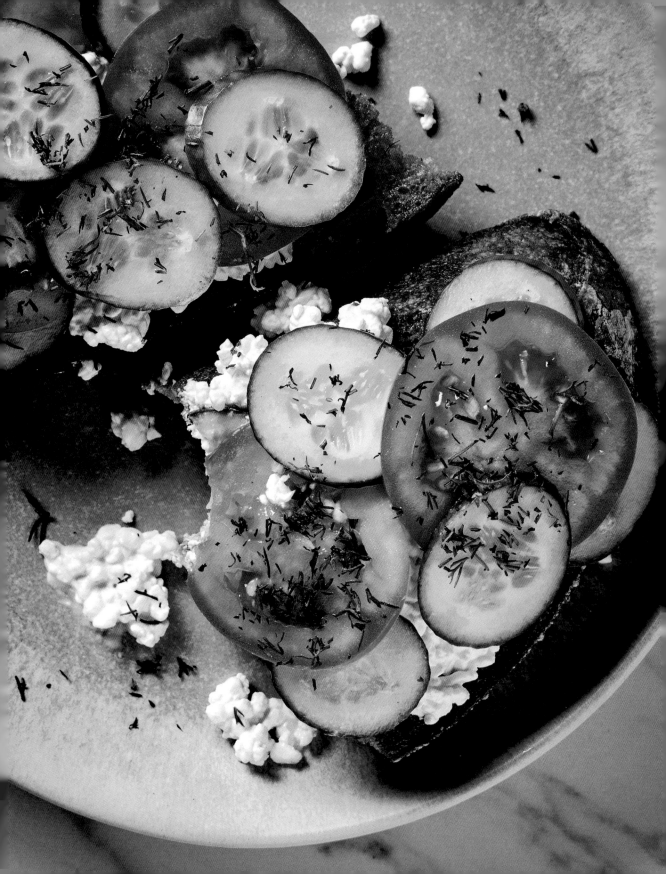

my favorite toast

I could eat this toast for every single meal and not grow tired of it. When you toast fresh bread in olive oil and season it with salt and garlic powder, it's a totally unique experience that lets the toppings shine more than a sandwich would. For this toast, the cottage cheese is creamy and filling, and the tomatoes and cucumbers add a refreshing crunch. Plus, there's a ton of protein to keep you full throughout the day. I eat this most often when I need a quick snack between meetings, and it's great if you're looking for something low-key with ingredients you already have. **SERVES 1 OR 2**

1 teaspoon extra virgin olive oil

1 or 2 slices fresh sourdough bread

Fine sea salt, to taste

Garlic powder, to taste

One 5-ounce container whole milk cottage cheese (I prefer Good Culture brand)

1 Roma tomato, cut into ½-inch slices

1 Persian cucumber, cut into ¼-inch slices

Freshly ground black pepper

Finely chopped fresh herbs (optional)

1. Heat the olive oil in a large skillet over medium-high heat. Pan-fry the bread until golden brown, 4 to 5 minutes per side. Remove the toast from the pan and season with salt and garlic powder.

2. Spread a thick layer of cottage cheese on the toasted bread. Cover with the sliced tomatoes and cucumbers and season with more salt and pepper to taste. Garnish with fresh herbs, if desired.

avocado & tomato toast

This recipe is just one example of how you can use the leftover small plates from the previous section to make a quick, delicious meal or snack. If I'm planning to make this toast in particular, I like to make the Tomato Salad (page 17) with those small, shiny cherry tomatoes I can often find at the market and cut them into quarters. I've also been known to chop up some scallions or herbs and add those to the tomatoes, so get creative based on what you have. **SERVES 1 OR 2**

1 teaspoon extra virgin olive oil

1 or 2 slices fresh sourdough bread

¼ teaspoon fine sea salt, plus more to taste

¼ teaspoon garlic powder, plus more to taste

1 ripe avocado

Freshly ground black pepper

Juice of ½ lemon (about 1½ tablespoons)

½ cup Tomato Salad (page 17), made with cherry tomatoes

1. Heat the olive oil in a large skillet over medium-high heat. Pan-fry the bread until golden brown, 4 to 5 minutes per side. Remove the toast from the pan and sprinkle with the salt and the garlic powder.

2. Halve, pit, and dice the avocado. Season with additional garlic powder, salt, a few turns of pepper, and a squeeze of lemon. Mash the avocado on top of the bread.

3. Spoon the tomato salad over the avocado and adjust the seasonings to taste.

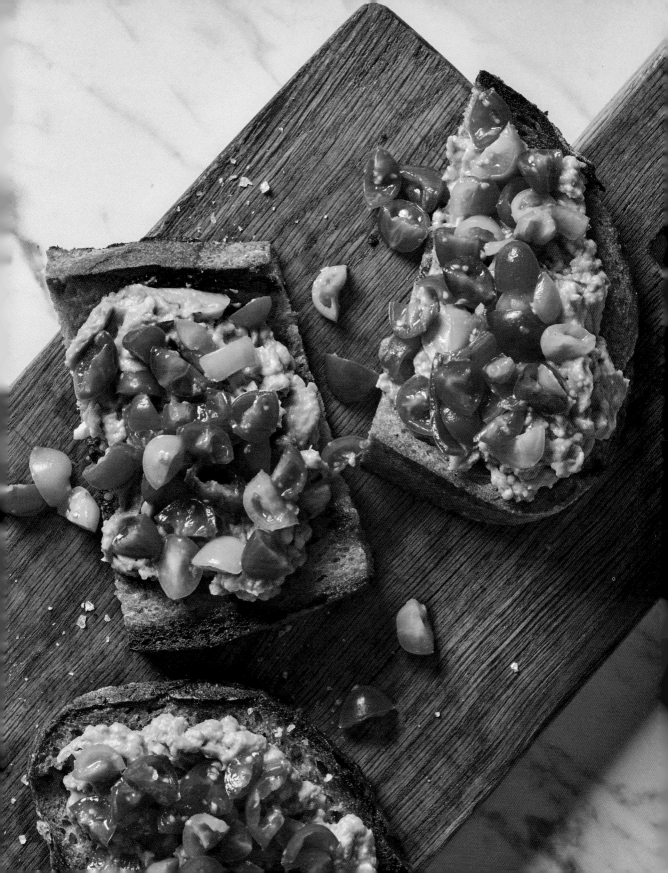

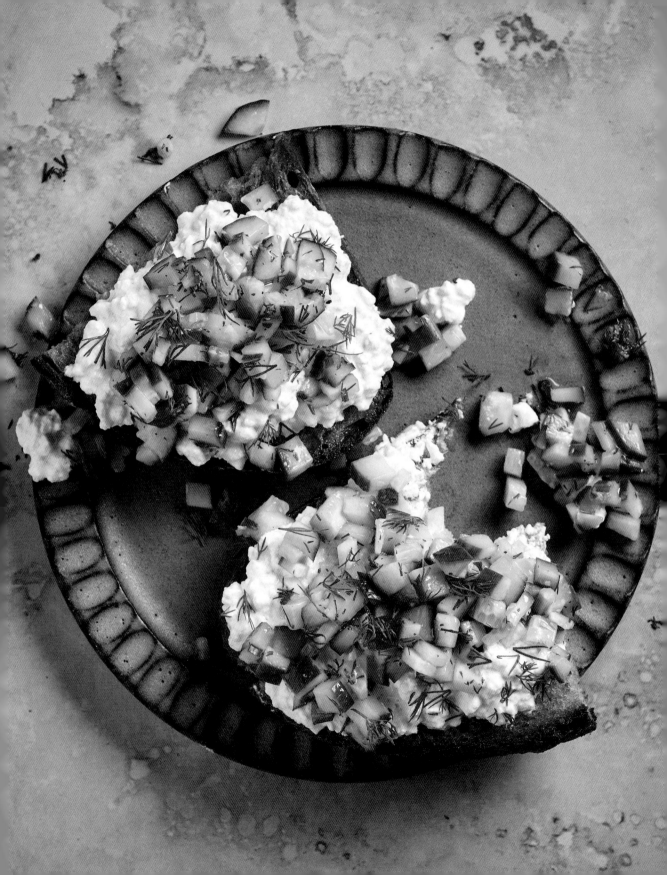

cucumber & cottage cheese toast

This salad reminds me of biting into a pickle in all the best ways, with refreshing herbs and a burst of acidity. The combination of fresh dill and garlic has an undeniable pickle quality to it, which here serves to enhance the sweet cucumber flavor while letting dill have its moment in the spotlight. It pairs so well with creamy cottage cheese and flavorful toast fried in olive oil that I'd happily eat this every day (and sometimes do). My mouth waters just thinking about it. **SERVES 2**

4 Persian cucumbers, cut into confetti-size pieces

2 tablespoons chopped fresh dill

Juice of 1 lemon (about 3 tablespoons)

3 tablespoons plus 1 teaspoon extra virgin olive oil

1 tablespoon white vinegar

1 garlic clove, grated with a Microplane

¼ teaspoon fine sea salt, plus more to taste

2 slices fresh sourdough bread

Garlic powder, to taste

1 cup whole milk cottage cheese

1. Place the cucumbers in a large bowl.

2. Whisk together the dill, lemon juice, 3 tablespoons of the olive oil, the vinegar, grated garlic, and salt in a small bowl, then pour over the cucumbers. Stir well to combine.

3. Heat the remaining 1 teaspoon olive oil in a large skillet over medium-high heat. Pan-fry the bread until golden brown, 4 to 5 minutes per side. Remove the toast from the pan and season with salt and garlic powder.

4. Spoon ½ cup of the cottage cheese over each piece of toast. Top with the cucumber salad.

note: It's important to serve this recipe immediately after you make it, so make sure you're ready to eat before you start—if it sits too long in the fridge, it will pickle!

mediterranean toast

Spooning leftover Mediterranean Chopped Salad (page 97) over a freshly toasted piece of bread spread with Roasted Garlic Dip (page 35) feels like going to a restaurant. Someone has already done all the hard work for you, even if it was you who finely chopped all those vegetables with love the day before. Sprinkle feta, fresh herbs, or seeds on top to make it really feel fancy, and you may never want to go out again. **SERVES 1 OR 2**

1 teaspoon extra virgin olive oil

1 or 2 slices fresh sourdough bread

Fine sea salt, to taste

Garlic powder, to taste

2 tablespoons Roasted Garlic Dip (page 35), or store-bought garlic dip or hummus

1 cup Mediterranean Chopped Salad (page 97)

Crumbled feta, for garnish

1. Heat the olive oil in a large skillet over medium-high heat. Pan-fry the bread until golden brown, 4 to 5 minutes per side. Remove the toast from the pan and season with salt and garlic powder.

2. Spread garlic dip over the toast.

3. Top with the chopped salad and garnish with feta.

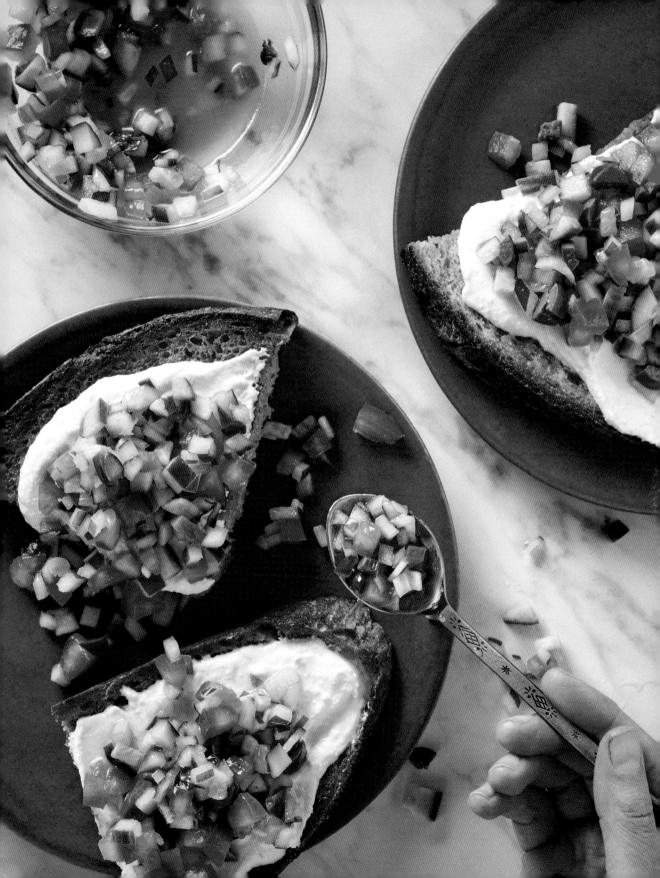

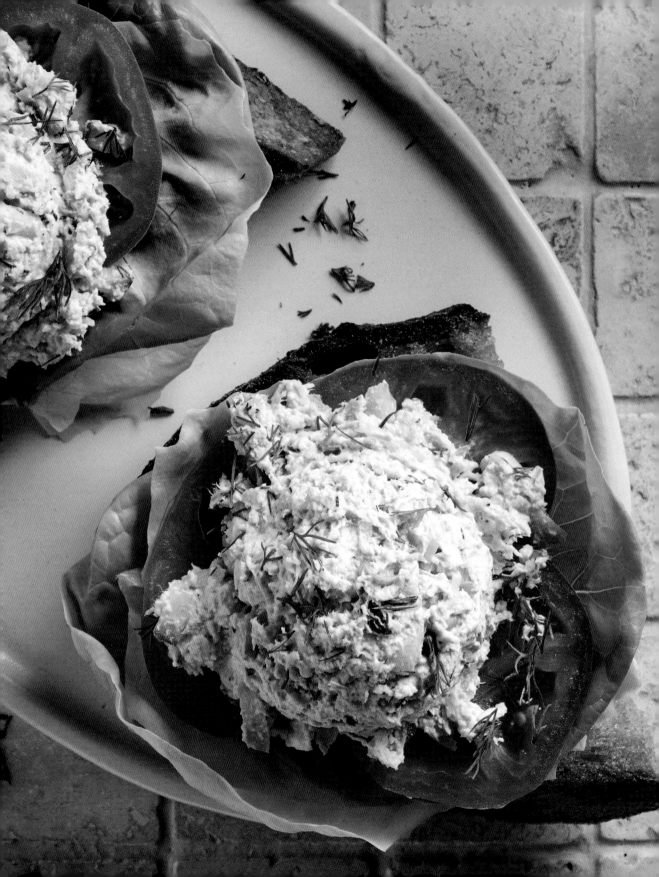

dilly chicken salad on toast

Crunchy, salty pickles are an incredible addition to so many meals. The acidity helps cut fattiness, and even a small amount adds so much flavor. Adding fresh dill and briny pickles to chicken salad takes it from ordinary to addictive. There's just the right amount of crunch from extra veggies (carrots, celery, and the pickles), and a tangy bite from the mustard. I prefer to serve it as an open-faced sandwich, since you get two sandwiches for the price of one—meaning more delicious bites and more variety. **MAKES 4 CUPS CHICKEN SALAD; SERVES 4 TO 6**

FOR THE SALAD

1 pound boneless, skinless chicken breasts, cooked using the Simple Grilled Chicken recipe (page 84), or you can use a rotisserie chicken

2 celery stalks, finely chopped

2 medium carrots, peeled and grated

2 scallions, trimmed, white and light green parts finely chopped

1 tablespoon chopped fresh dill

3 small dill pickles or ½ large dill pickle, finely chopped

FOR THE DRESSING

Juice of 2 lemons (about ⅓ cup)

⅓ cup mayonnaise

¼ cup Dijon mustard

1 tablespoon pickle juice

1 large garlic clove, minced

1 teaspoon garlic powder

½ teaspoon fine sea salt

¼ teaspoon freshly ground black pepper

FOR THE TOAST

1 teaspoon extra virgin olive oil

4 to 6 slices fresh sourdough bread

Lettuce, to serve

Tomato slices, to serve

Fresh dill, chopped, for garnish

1. MAKE THE CHICKEN SALAD: Add the chicken to the bowl of a stand mixer fitted with the paddle attachment. Shred the chicken on medium speed. If you don't have a stand mixer, place the chicken in a large bowl and shred with a hand mixer, or simply shred with two forks.

2. Mix in the celery, carrots, scallions, dill, and pickles on low to combine.

3. MAKE THE DRESSING: Whisk together the lemon juice, mayonnaise, mustard, pickle juice, garlic, garlic powder, salt, and pepper in a small bowl.

4. Combine the dressing with the chicken mixture.

5. PREPARE THE TOAST: Heat the olive oil in a large skillet over medium-high heat. Pan-fry the bread until golden brown, 4 to 5 minutes per side. Remove the toast from the pan.

6. Scoop the chicken salad onto the bread with the lettuce and tomato and serve open-faced. Garnish with fresh dill.

green goddess toast

If you think you don't like leftovers, this is the recipe that will change your mind. If you've ever made the Green Goddess Salad (page 98), you know it feeds a crowd—and sometimes, eating it over and over again can get repetitive. I get it! This toast is on constant rotation in our house, elevating humble avocado toast with fresh veggies and a nice Jammy Egg (page 22) or sunny-side up egg on top. The leftovers are just as good as the fresh salad, if not better. If you don't have leftover Green Goddess, it works with just about any other salad you love. **SERVES 1 OR 2**

2 teaspoons extra virgin olive oil

2 large eggs

Flaky sea salt

Freshly ground black pepper

1 or 2 slices fresh sourdough bread

1 garlic clove, cut in half

1 avocado, thinly sliced

1 cup Green Goddess Salad (page 98)

1. Heat 1 teaspoon of the olive oil in a nonstick pan over medium heat.

2. Crack the eggs into the hot pan. Cover the pan and cook for 2 to 3 minutes, until the whites are cooked through. Season with salt and pepper and remove from the heat.

3. Heat the remaining 1 teaspoon olive oil in a large skillet over medium-high heat. Pan-fry the bread until golden brown, 4 to 5 minutes per side. Remove the toast from the pan.

4. Rub the garlic across the toast.

5. Cover the toast with the avocado slices.

6. Add a layer of the Green Goddess Salad.

7. Place the eggs over the toast and sprinkle with flaky sea salt.

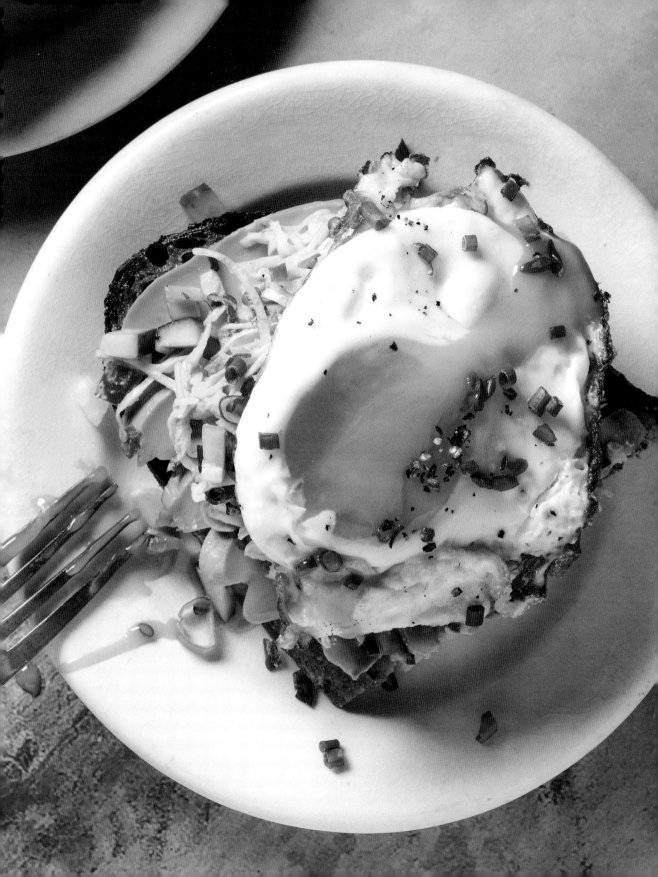

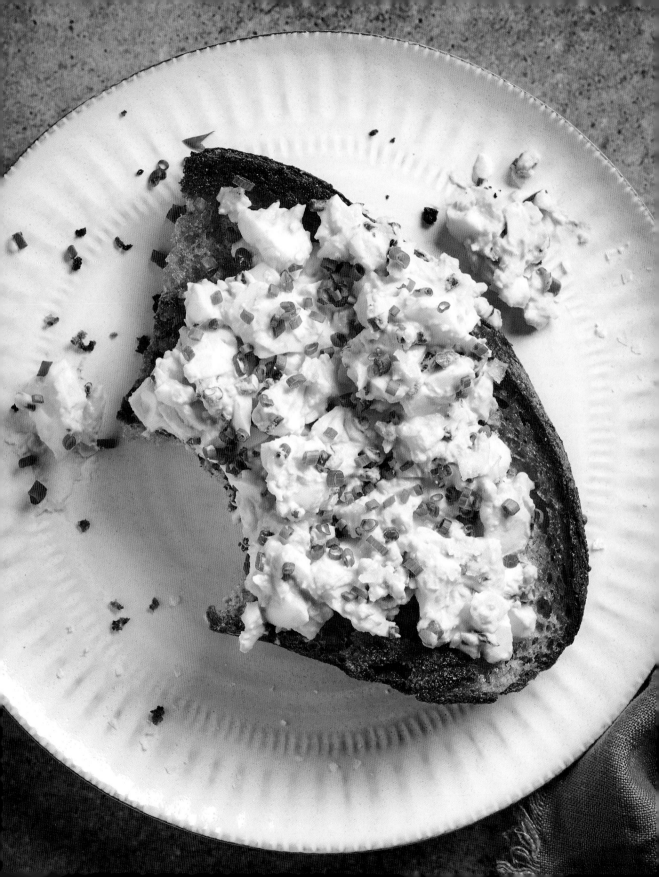

egg salad toast

One of the things I love about social media is that it gives me the opportunity to learn firsthand what people love to eat. This egg salad is fast and easy to make for a filling midday meal and has a deliciously creamy, tangy flavor. Whenever I post an egg salad on TikTok, people literally eat it up and comment on how much they love this classic. Sometimes, I'll combine it with potatoes or tuna salad for a more filling meal (and for more variety), but egg salad alone on a crunchy piece of toast is so satisfying. I like to mash the egg yolks together with the dressing ingredients, then fold the egg whites in so every bite is packed with flavor. **SERVES 1 OR 2**

10 large brown eggs (they're easier to peel)

2 tablespoons mayonnaise

1 tablespoon German mustard

¼ teaspoon fine sea salt

2 tablespoons pickle juice

Juice of ¼ lemon (about 2 teaspoons)

¼ cup chopped fresh chives

1 teaspoon extra virgin olive oil

1 or 2 slices fresh sourdough bread

Garlic powder, to taste

1. Bring a large pot of water to boil over high heat. Add the eggs and cook, uncovered, for 12 minutes. While the eggs cook, prepare an ice bath.

2. When the eggs are finished cooking, place them in the ice bath for at least 1 minute to cool. Peel the eggs and rinse off any excess pieces of shell.

3. Using two mixing bowls, separate the egg whites from the egg yolks.

4. Mash the yolks together with the mayonnaise, mustard, salt, pickle juice, lemon juice, and 2 tablespoons cold water. It should form a loose paste.

5. Cut the egg whites into bite-size pieces and add them to the bowl with the yolk dressing.

6. Add the chives and stir well to combine.

7. Heat the olive oil in a large skillet over medium-high heat. Pan-fry the bread until golden brown, 4 to 5 minutes per side. Remove the toast from the pan.

8. Sprinkle with garlic powder and spoon the egg salad on top. Store any leftover egg salad in an airtight container in the fridge for up to 3 days.

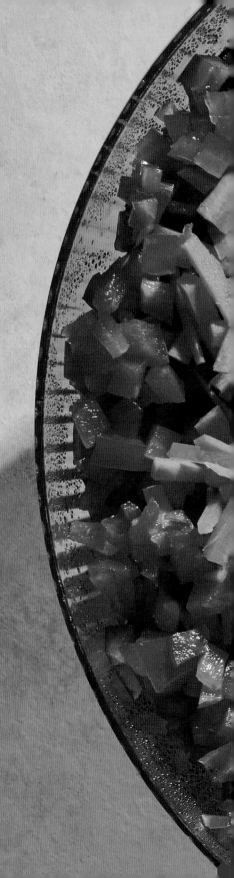

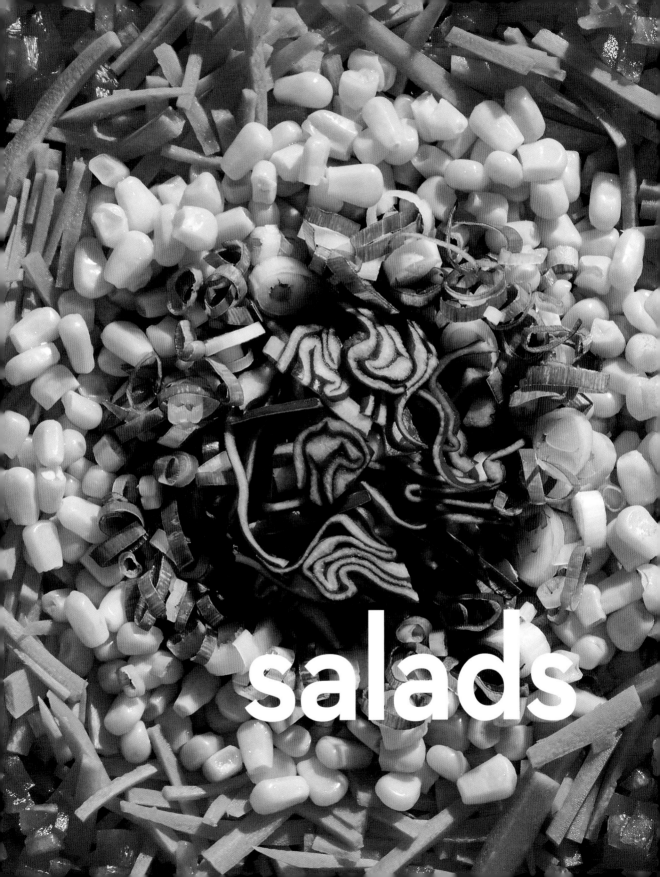

salads

Every salad recipe in this book has one thing in common: They're designed to give you the perfect bite. This is in large part what makes eating salads enjoyable, because you get a little bit of everything on your fork at once. That's why I chop my vegetables so finely and why none of these salads would dare be underdressed. With the right ratio of nourishing greens, crunch, herbs, and color, every salad becomes a mouthwatering meal that you'll dream about day and night, just like I do.

It's no secret I'm obsessed with the perfect bite—just look at Baked by Melissa, the company I cofounded fifteen-plus years ago and still run today. Baked by Melissa has one product: a bite-size treat with the perfect ratio of flavor in each and every bite. I see the bite-size cupcake as my vessel for flavor. Much like my salads, the components never change, with a base of cake, some sort of delicious stuffing, and a topping that not only complements the cupcake's flavor but also makes it look beautiful. One bite of a Baked by Melissa cupcake and the taste instantly transports you to a nostalgic moment. When I create salad recipes, my creative process is quite similar to that of flavor development at Baked by Melissa. These recipes don't use groundbreaking ingredients or flavor combinations you've never seen before. Just like with my cupcakes, I take familiar, classic, and often nostalgic flavor profiles and put my own spin on them to provide you with the perfect bite.

> **"Every salad recipe in this book has one thing in common: They're designed to give you the perfect bite."**

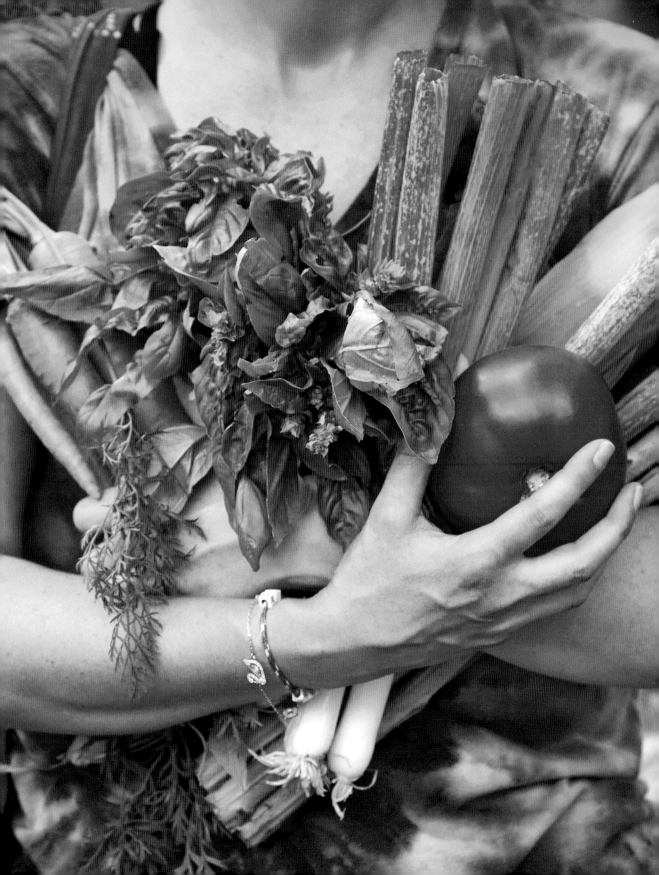

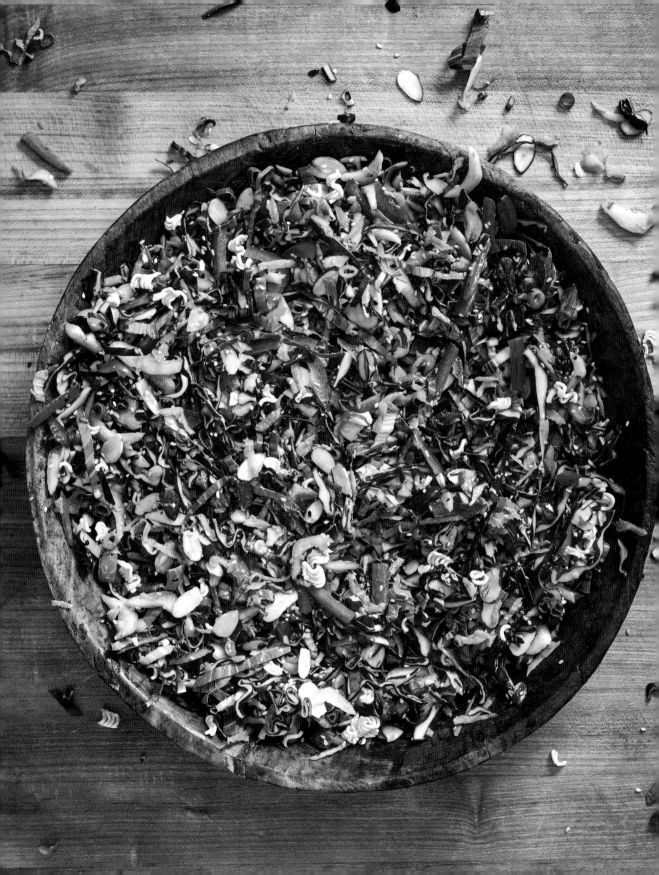

crunchy ramen slaw with grilled ribeye

My mom made a variation of this salad throughout my whole childhood. Maybe yours did, too. For me, it's one of the oldest recipes in this book, though I did update it by making a few adjustments to my mom's original recipe. I swapped honey for sugar, olive oil for canola, and added a few more colored veggies into the mix. But it still brings back fond memories of sitting with my family around the dinner table.

The most fun part of this salad is using the instant ramen that you can find at any grocery store, crumbling the block of noodles into pieces and whisking the seasoning packet into the dressing. Instant ramen is super affordable, and it's a great way to get kids involved in the kitchen (mine love to bang the ramen on the counter). Make this a staple in your house for gatherings or weeknight meals—trust me, the memories are worth it.

SERVES 8

3 baby bok choy, cut into ¼-inch pieces

2 cups finely shredded red cabbage

2 medium carrots, peeled and grated

1 red bell pepper, thinly sliced and cut into 1-inch lengths

1 bunch scallions, trimmed, white and light green parts cut into ¼-inch slices

½ cup sliced almonds

2 tablespoons sesame seeds

1 package ramen noodles, broken into small pieces

Sliced Grilled Ribeye, to serve (recipe follows)

1. Combine the bok choy, cabbage, carrots, red pepper, and scallions in a large bowl; cover and chill while you make the rest of the salad.

2. MAKE THE DRESSING: Whisk together the ramen seasoning packet, sesame oil, vinegar, olive oil, lemon juice, salt, honey, garlic, and pepper in a small bowl and refrigerate until cold.

3. Heat a pan over medium heat and add the sliced almonds and sesame seeds. Cook, tossing occasionally, until the almonds and seeds are fragrant and golden brown, 3 to 5 minutes.

4. Remove the salad from the refrigerator. Top with the toasted almonds, sesame seeds, and the broken ramen noodles. Pour the dressing over the salad and mix well to evenly coat.

(continued)

FOR THE DRESSING

Beef-flavored ramen seasoning packet

3 tablespoons toasted sesame oil

3 tablespoons white vinegar

⅓ cup extra virgin olive oil

Juice of 1 lemon (about 3 tablespoons)

1 teaspoon fine sea salt

1 teaspoon honey

1 garlic clove, grated with a Microplane

½ teaspoon freshly ground black pepper

5. Serve with sliced grilled ribeye. This is best enjoyed the day you make it, so if you don't think you'll eat it all, save a portion of dressing and a portion of undressed salad in airtight containers in the fridge for up to 3 days.

note: If you don't eat red meat or want to cut costs, the Simple Grilled Chicken (page 84) or Grilled Soy Tofu (page 93) work well, too.

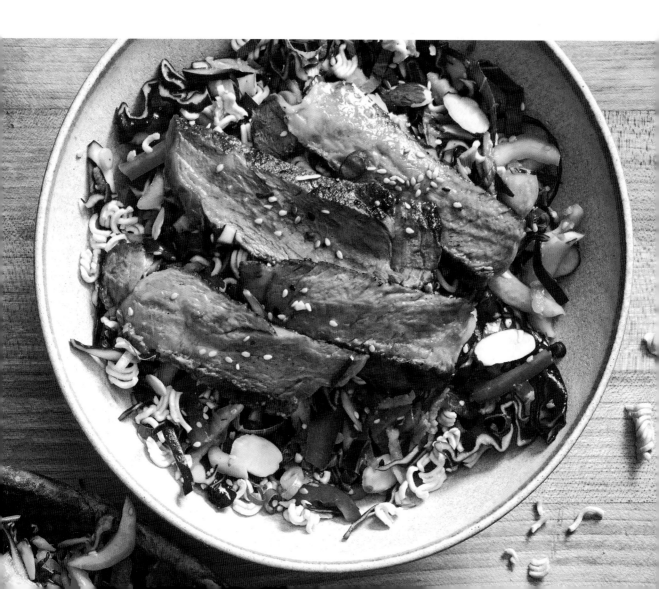

sliced grilled ribeye Everyone in my family loves a good ribeye, even my kids. It's my favorite cut of beef, with delicious flavor from the ribbons of fat that also allow you to cook it quickly. Although it can be expensive, I do find that a good ribeye is the perfect complement to any salad you want to enjoy as a meal, the Crunchy Ramen Slaw included. It's so tender, which lends itself to the perfect bite. **SERVES 4**

1 tablespoon extra virgin olive oil

Two 1¼-pound grass-fed, bone-in ribeye steaks, at room temperature

1 teaspoon fine sea salt

1 teaspoon freshly ground black pepper

1. Heat the olive oil in a cast-iron skillet on the stove over medium-high heat. Preheat the oven to 275°F.

2. Pat the steaks dry with a paper towel and season liberally with the salt and pepper.

3. Once the skillet is hot, add the ribeyes. Sear for 1 to 2 minutes on each side, depending on how thick they are. If they're less than 1 inch thick, cook for 1 minute; if they're 1½ inches, sear for 2 minutes. This will give them a crispy, delicious crust.

4. Once the steaks are seared, transfer the skillet to the oven. Cook for 18 to 20 minutes, again depending on the thickness of the steaks. If you prefer your steak medium-rare, let them reach an internal temperature of 130°F. For a medium steak, let them cook until they're around 135°F. Consider that the temperature will continue to rise after you remove the steaks from the oven, and will likely be a few degrees higher when you slice it.

5. Remove the steak from the pan and let rest for 10 to 15 minutes. Slice the meat against the grain into ½-inch pieces and use to top your favorite salad. Store any leftovers in an airtight container in the fridge for up to 3 days.

italian chopped salad

I grew up in northern New Jersey, where old-school Italian restaurants with checkered tablecloths line every block. This salad was inspired by the chef salads at those restaurants, with roasted red peppers, salami, and fresh mutz (that's how we say "mozzarella" in New Jersey). I love that this variation includes so many pantry staples, making it easy to whip up. Everything in the salad should be cut into equal ¼-inch to ½-inch pieces to get the perfect bite, and since the base of this salad is romaine, wait to dress it until right before you serve so it doesn't get soggy. **SERVES 4 TO 6**

2 bunches romaine lettuce, cut into ¼-inch pieces

5 Persian cucumbers, finely chopped

1 bunch scallions, trimmed, light green and white parts cut into ¼-inch slices

2 roasted red peppers, drained, thinly sliced, and cut into ½-inch pieces

¼ cup Castelvetrano olives, finely chopped

One 15-ounce can chickpeas, drained and rinsed

5 to 6 hearts of palm, drained and finely chopped

One 6.5-ounce jar artichoke hearts marinated in oil, drained and finely chopped

½ cup grape tomatoes, cut in half

1 cup roughly chopped fresh mozzarella

FOR THE ITALIAN VINAIGRETTE

¼ cup red wine vinegar

⅓ cup extra virgin olive oil

Juice of 2 lemons (about ⅓ cup)

1 heaping teaspoon dried oregano

½ teaspoon garlic powder

½ teaspoon onion powder

1 heaping teaspoon chopped fresh parsley

2 large garlic cloves, grated with a Microplane

1 teaspoon fine sea salt

2 tablespoons nutritional yeast

¼ teaspoon freshly ground black pepper

1. Combine the romaine, cucumbers, scallions, roasted red peppers, olives, chickpeas, hearts of palm, artichoke hearts, tomatoes, and mozzarella in a large bowl.

2. MAKE THE VINAIGRETTE: Add the vinegar, olive oil, lemon juice, oregano, garlic powder, onion powder, parsley, grated garlic, salt, nutritional yeast, and pepper to a small bowl and whisk until fully combined.

3. Pour the dressing over the vegetables and toss to get each and every bite evenly covered. Serve immediately.

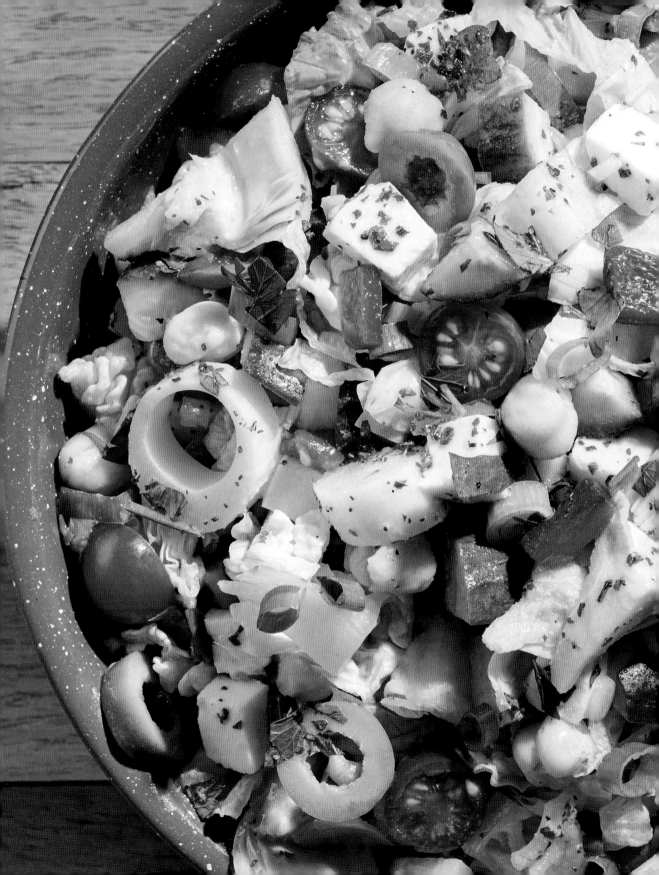

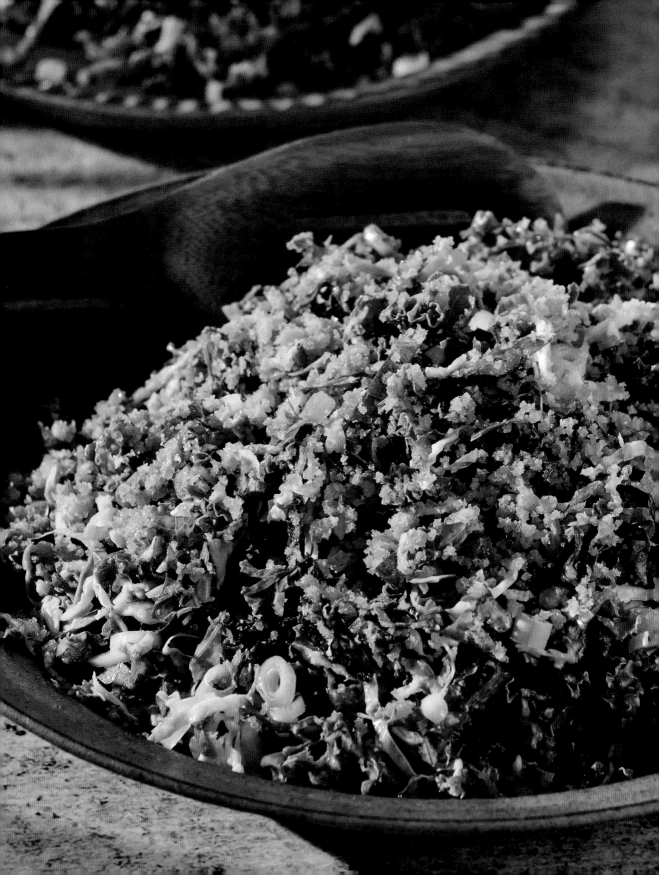

kale caesar with garlicky panko and simple salmon

When I was a kid, I loved ordering a Caesar salad anytime it was on the menu. Like Joe's Honey Chicken Salad (page 75), it's a segue salad, with big bites of romaine serving as a vessel for cheesy, creamy flavor.

Traditional Caesar dressing includes egg, Worcestershire sauce, anchovies, and Parmesan, resulting in a crowd-pleasing, flavorful dressing. To make it vegan, I use hummus and nutritional yeast for creaminess, and the lemon juice and capers mimic the zing of anchovies. Instead of croutons, I use crunchy, garlicky panko, which when sprinkled over the kale softens the salad a bit and creates forkfuls of crunchy bites evenly covered in a creamy dressing—just like those Caesars I used to love as a kid. **SERVES 4 TO 6**

FOR THE SIMPLE SALMON

Two 6-ounce organic salmon fillets

Juice of 1 lemon (about 3 tablespoons)

½ teaspoon fine sea salt

2 tablespoons extra virgin olive oil

1 garlic clove, grated with a Microplane

Freshly ground black pepper

FOR THE SALAD

1 bunch kale (about ½ pound), stems removed, leaves sliced into thin ribbons (see page 251)

1 pound Brussels sprouts, trimmed and shredded with a mandoline

3 to 4 scallions, trimmed, white and light green parts cut into ¼-inch slices

Vegan Caesar Dressing (recipe follows)

Garlicky Panko, for topping (recipe follows)

1. MAKE THE SALMON: If using an oven, line a baking sheet with parchment paper. If using an air fryer, line the air fryer basket with parchment paper. Preheat the oven or air fryer to 400°F.

2. Pat the salmon dry with a paper towel and place it on the prepared baking sheet or in the prepared air fryer basket. Cover with the lemon juice and sprinkle with the salt.

3. Whisk together the olive oil and garlic in a small bowl. Brush the mixture over the salmon and bake for 10 to 15 minutes, until it flakes easily with a fork.

4. While the salmon cooks, combine the kale, Brussels sprouts, and scallions in a large bowl.

5. Season the salmon with freshly ground black pepper.

6. Pour the vegan Caesar dressing over the salad and toss to combine.

7. Top with garlicky panko and salmon.

(continued)

vegan caesar dressing

MAKES ABOUT 1¼ CUPS DRESSING

¼ cup plain hummus

1 teaspoon Dijon mustard

Juice of 2 lemons (about ⅓ cup)

2 garlic cloves, grated with a
Microplane

2 tablespoons capers packed
in brine, finely chopped, plus
1 tablespoon brine

1 teaspoon fine sea salt

3 tablespoons extra virgin olive oil

⅓ cup nutritional yeast

Whisk together the hummus, mustard, lemon juice, garlic, capers, caper brine, salt, olive oil, and nutritional yeast in a small bowl until well combined.

garlicky panko

MAKES 1 CUP

3 tablespoons extra virgin olive oil

1 cup panko breadcrumbs

½ teaspoon fine sea salt

2 garlic cloves

1. Heat the olive oil in a medium skillet over medium heat.

2. Add the panko to the pan and stir so that the breadcrumbs are coated in the oil. Season with the salt. Grate the garlic into the pan with a Microplane and stir everything together.

3. Toast the breadcrumbs, stirring occasionally, until golden brown, 4 to 5 minutes. Use as a salad or pasta topping.

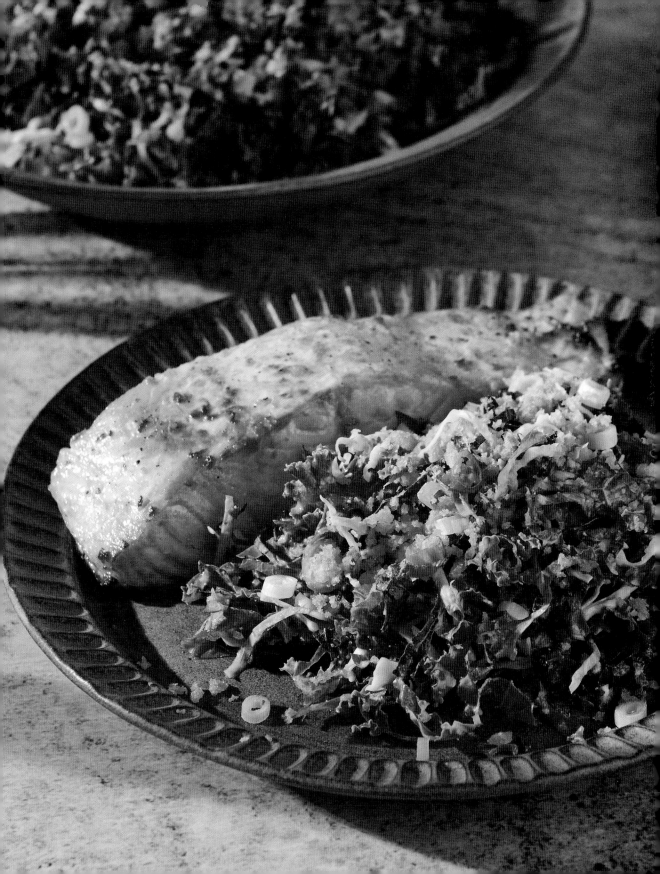

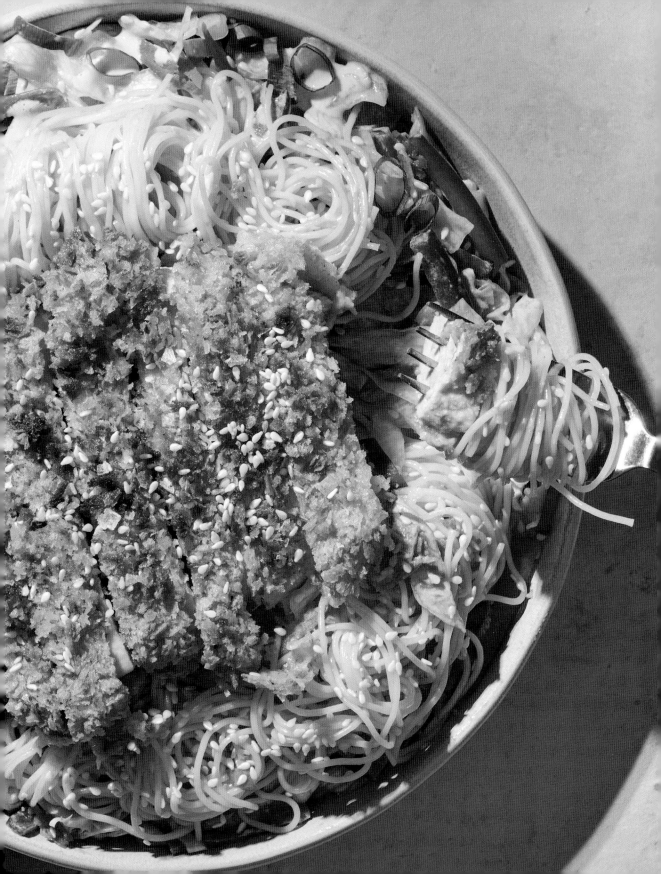

joe's honey chicken salad

When I was a teenager, mall culture was at its peak. Going to Garden State Plaza Mall after school or on weekends was a pretty common activity for us; my friends and I would walk around, and our parents would give us money to have lunch while we were there.

My best friend and I always went to Joe's American Bar & Grill, and, without fail, I would always order the honey chicken salad, which inspired this recipe. I think it was one of my segue salads, because it's a great entry point for people who claim not to love salads. As a kid, I loved that it had chicken fingers and pasta—it's a very basic lettuce-based salad with hearty toppings, a little sesame, and a little honey. I highly recommend making it for kids to get them excited about salad and vegetables. This recipe calls for air fryer chicken, but you can use a cutlet or any other protein to make it your own. I can still taste Joe's salad if I close my eyes and think back to those days, and this recipe takes me there. I mean, what's better than a salad filled with crispy chicken and pasta? **SERVES 4 TO 6**

1 head iceberg lettuce, sliced into thin ribbons

1 bunch scallions, trimmed, white and light green parts cut into ¼-inch slices

1 red bell pepper, thinly sliced and cut into 1 inch pieces

2 carrots, peeled and grated

One 8-ounce package angel hair pasta, cooked according to package directions and cooled

1 tablespoon toasted sesame oil

2 tablespoons sesame seeds, plus more for garnish

Fine sea salt

3 Crispy Air Fryer Chicken cutlets (recipe follows), for serving

FOR THE DRESSING

⅓ cup mayonnaise

⅓ cup Dijon mustard

2 tablespoons honey

1 teaspoon fine sea salt

Juice of ½ lemon (about 1½ tablespoons)

1. Combine the iceberg, scallions, red pepper, and carrots in a large bowl.

2. MAKE THE DRESSING: Whisk together the mayo, mustard, honey, salt, and lemon juice in a small bowl until smooth.

3. Pour the dressing over the iceberg mix and toss to evenly coat.

4. In a separate bowl, coat the cooked angel hair in the sesame oil and sprinkle with the sesame seeds. Season with salt and add to the salad. Toss gently to combine.

5. Portion out each serving in a bowl and top with the crispy chicken. Garnish with sesame seeds.

(continued)

crispy air fryer chicken

MAKES 3 CUTLETS

3 boneless, skinless chicken breasts

Juice of ½ lemon (about 1½ tablespoons), plus more for serving

½ teaspoon fine sea salt, plus more to taste

1 large egg, beaten

½ cup panko breadcrumbs

⅓ cup all-purpose flour

¼ teaspoon freshly ground black pepper

½ teaspoon garlic powder

½ teaspoon sweet paprika with oil

Extra virgin olive oil spray

1. Line the air fryer basket with parchment paper. Preheat the air fryer to 350°F.

2. If needed, pound the chicken so it's about ½ inch thick. Squeeze the lemon over the chicken and season with ¼ teaspoon of the salt.

3. Organize three bowls: one with the egg, one with the breadcrumbs, and one with the flour. Add the remaining ¼ teaspoon salt, the pepper, garlic powder, and paprika to the flour and stir to combine.

4. Dredge the chicken in the flour, then the egg, then the panko, making sure that the chicken is fully coated. Repeat with each breast.

5. Place the chicken in the prepared air fryer basket and spray each side of the chicken with olive oil. Bake for about 10 minutes, or until the juices run clear and the chicken is golden.

6. Season with salt and a squeeze of lemon juice.

vegan taco salad

Creating incredible vegan meals that are as nutritious as they are delicious requires a bit of extra thought and creativity, but it's so worth it. This salad is everything I love about a classic taco salad, from the flavorful protein to the bright herbs, but with even more fresh ingredients. You can use any of the small plates from this book as toppings (especially the tomato and avocado salads; see pages 17 and 21), or you can make this with individual ingredients like I did here. This recipe is super flexible, so you can make tacos for your kids and a salad for yourself while enjoying a fun meal together. **SERVES 4 TO 6**

1 head iceberg lettuce, cut into ¼-inch pieces

3 Persian cucumbers, cut into confetti-size pieces

1 red bell pepper, thinly sliced then cut into ½-inch pieces

One 15-ounce can black beans, drained and rinsed

1 bunch scallions, trimmed, light green and white parts cut into ¼-inch slices

2 Roma tomatoes, finely chopped

1 ripe avocado, diced

½ cup pickled red onions (see page 262)

Crispy Taco Tofu (recipe follows)

½ cup crushed tortilla chips

FOR THE DRESSING

Juice of 2 lemons (about ⅓ cup)

3 tablespoons extra virgin olive oil

1½ tablespoons (or a healthy splash) white vinegar

2 large garlic cloves, minced

¾ teaspoon fine sea salt

1. Place the lettuce in a large bowl. To make the dressing, whisk together the lemon juice, olive oil, vinegar, garlic, and salt. Pour over the iceberg and toss to combine.

2. Add the cucumbers, red pepper, beans, scallions, and tomatoes and stir to combine.

3. Top with the avocado, pickled red onions, and tofu. Garnish with the crushed tortilla chips.

   note: The Crispy Taco Tofu in this recipe requires freezing overnight, so make sure you prep that the day before you plan to eat this!

   (continued)

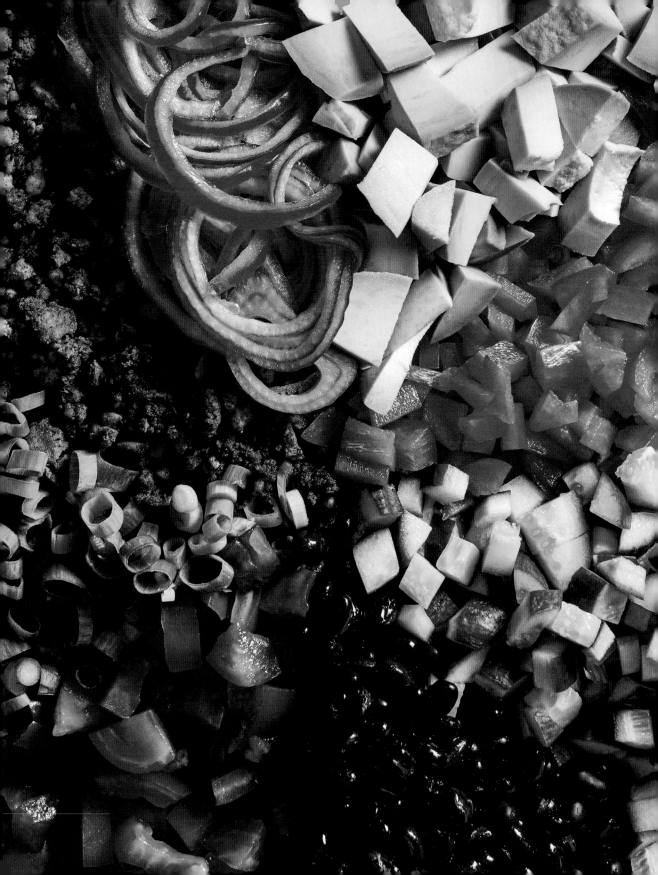

crispy taco tofu

SERVES 4

1 block extra-firm tofu

3 tablespoons avocado oil

2 tablespoons taco seasoning (I like Garden of Eatin')

Fine sea salt

1. Drain the tofu and place in an airtight container or freezer-safe bag. Freeze the tofu overnight, or for at least 8 hours so it freezes fully.

2. Let the tofu thaw in a strainer set over a bowl to get rid of excess water. Once it's fully thawed, press out any remaining excess water. Now, it should crumble easily. With your hands, break the tofu into small pieces over a tea towel. If using an air fryer, line the air fryer basket with parchment paper. If using an oven, line a baking sheet with parchment paper. Preheat the air fryer to 350°F or the oven to 375°F.

3. Place the tofu in a bowl and toss with the avocado oil and taco seasoning. Wait to salt until it's finished cooking, since different taco seasonings have different levels of salt.

4. Arrange the tofu in a single layer in the prepared air fryer basket or on the prepared baking sheet. Air-fry the tofu until crispy, 20 to 30 minutes, stirring about halfway through. If using the oven bake for 25 to 35 minutes, stirring occasionally.

5. Salt to taste and serve on salad or in tacos.

kale cobb salad with crispy shallots

I've always loved a good Cobb salad. I remember loving them even as a kid because they were so approachable and I had the ability to easily remove things I didn't like (like blue cheese). Every time I go to Bubby's in Tribeca, I order the Cobb with cheddar cheese. Now, I appreciate the versatility of Cobbs: They can be totally adapted based on what you have in your fridge. I always use my miso vinaigrette for it, because it goes so well with any green (especially hearty kale) *and* any topping you feel like throwing on top. Go ahead, turn those leftovers into a salad. **SERVES 4 TO 6**

1 bunch kale (about ½ pound), stems removed, leaves sliced into thin ribbons (see page 251)

1 avocado, diced

1 cup diced fresh mozzarella

1 pint cherry tomatoes, halved

1 bunch scallions, trimmed, white and light green parts cut into ¼-inch slices

1½ cups diced Simple Grilled Chicken (page 84)

FOR THE VINAIGRETTE

¼ cup red wine vinegar

1 tablespoon dried oregano

½ teaspoon fine sea salt

1 teaspoon garlic powder

Juice of 2 lemons (about ⅓ cup)

⅓ cup nutritional yeast

3 tablespoons white miso paste

2 garlic cloves, grated with a Microplane

⅓ cup extra virgin olive oil

FOR THE CRISPY SHALLOTS

2 shallots, halved and thinly sliced

¼ cup all-purpose flour

Fine sea salt and freshly ground black pepper

2 tablespoons avocado oil

1. Combine the kale, avocado, mozzarella, cherry tomatoes, scallions, and chicken in a large bowl.

2. MAKE THE VINAIGRETTE: Whisk together the vinegar, oregano, salt, garlic powder, lemon juice, nutritional yeast, miso, and grated garlic. Drizzle in the oil and continuously whisk until the vinaigrette emulsifies. (Tip: Place the bowl over a tea towel to keep it stable while you whisk in the oil.)

3. MAKE THE CRISPY SHALLOTS: In a medium bowl, toss together the shallots and flour until fully coated. Season generously with salt and pepper. In a large skillet over medium-high heat, heat the avocado oil until shimmering. Fry the shallots until crispy and caramelized, 7 to 8 minutes. Remove the shallots from the pan with a slotted spoon to drain any excess oil and place them on a plate lined with a paper towel.

4. Pour the vinaigrette over the salad and toss to evenly coat.

5. Top with the crispy shallots and serve.

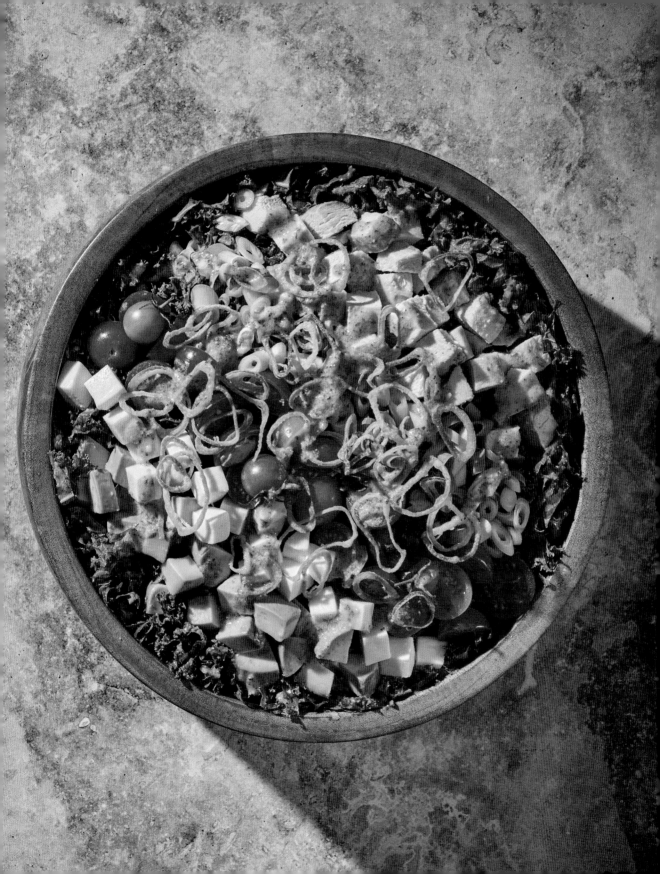

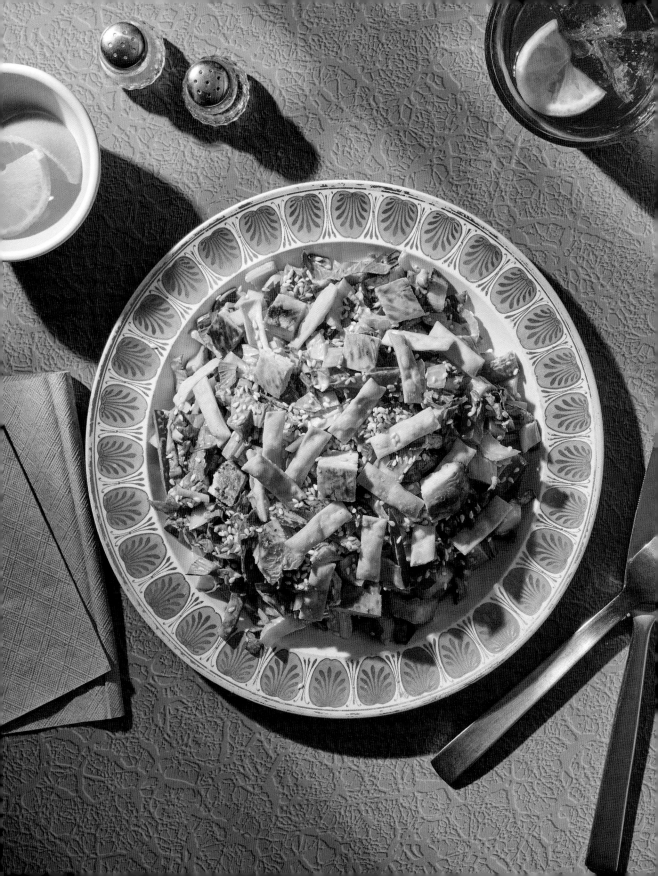

coffee shop sesame chicken salad

If you lived in or visited New York anytime from the '90s to 2018, you may have heard of the Coffee Shop. Its emblematic narrow neon sign beckoned everyone around Union Square, whether farmers' market shoppers, late-night bar crawlers, or the ladies on *Sex and the City*, all coming to see and be seen. But I myself was never in it to see or be seen—I was in it for the salads, and this is one I still dream about.

To be clear, this is my attempt to re-create the iconic salad I loved so much and relive some of my favorite memories. This salad is so good that I left my twenty-second birthday party early to pick up a few to-go for me and my friends. The salads were delicious, filled with crunchy bok choy and bell pepper, juicy chicken, and the most delectable creamy miso-ginger vinaigrette. The Coffee Shop unfortunately shuttered a few years ago, but one bite of this salad will take you back to its glory days or make you wish you'd had a chance to visit. **SERVES 4**

FOR THE CREAMY MISO-GINGER VINAIGRETTE

3 garlic cloves

One 1-inch knob fresh ginger, peeled (about 2 teaspoons grated ginger)

¼ cup toasted sesame oil

¼ cup avocado oil or other neutral oil

2 tablespoons white miso paste

2 tablespoons rice vinegar

Juice of 2 lemons (about ⅓ cup)

¼ cup nutritional yeast

1 teaspoon fine sea salt

FOR THE SALAD

2 large bunches bok choy, chopped

1 cup fresh spinach, chopped

½ red bell pepper, thinly sliced then cut into 1-inch pieces

Simple Grilled Chicken (recipe follows)

Toasted sesame seeds, to garnish

Store-bought wonton strips, to garnish

1. Add the garlic, ginger, sesame oil, avocado oil, miso, rice vinegar, lemon juice, nutritional yeast, and salt to a blender and process until smooth.

2. Combine the bok choy, spinach, and red pepper in a large bowl. Dice the grilled chicken and add it to the bowl. Pour the dressing over the veggies and toss gently until evenly coated.

3. Portion the salad out into bowls and garnish with sesame seeds and crunchy wonton strips.

(continued)

simple grilled chicken

SERVES 4

2 tablespoons avocado oil

1 teaspoon fine sea salt

1 teaspoon dried oregano

1 teaspoon garlic powder

¼ teaspoon freshly ground black pepper

Juice of 1 lemon (about 3 tablespoons)

4 boneless, skinless chicken breasts (1 pound), at room temperature

1. Whisk together the avocado oil, salt, oregano, garlic powder, pepper, and lemon juice in a small bowl to create a marinade.

2. Place the chicken on a large plate and cover completely with the marinade.

3. Heat a grill pan (or another nonstick pan) over medium-high heat. Carefully place the chicken in the pan with tongs. Pro tip: Position the biggest part of the breast toward the middle part of the pan, where the heat is. Don't crowd the chicken!

4. Cook for 5 minutes on each side (it should cleanly come off the pan when it's ready to flip). The chicken should reach an internal temperature of 165°F when it's fully cooked.

5. Remove the chicken to a plate and let rest for several minutes before dicing and adding to your salad.

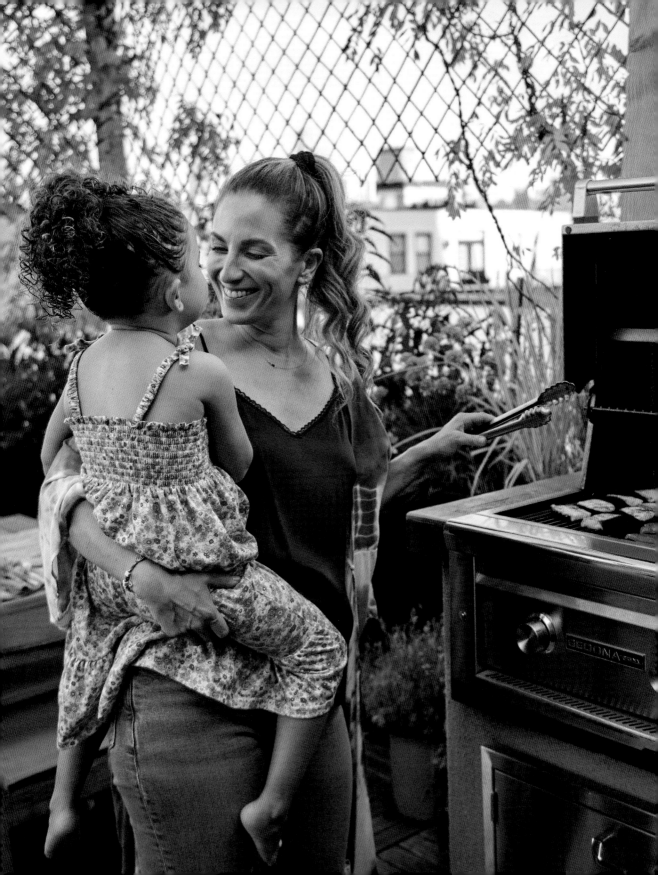

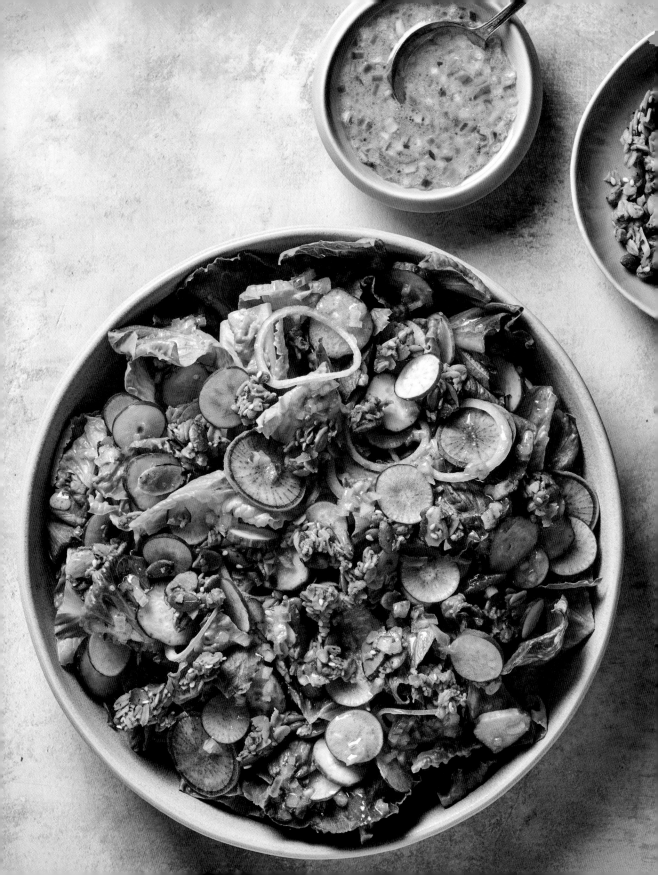

little gem & savory granola salad

little gem & savory granola salad If there is a little gem salad on the menu at a restaurant, I'm ordering it. You're almost guaranteed to receive a green, crunchy, yet simple salad with a dressing that won't disappoint. The countless little gem salads I've ordered in New York City (and beyond!) are absolutely the inspiration for this salad. This salad might seem simple to the naked eye, but sometimes it's the most perfect and seemingly simple things that require the most love and attention. The vibrant shallot vinaigrette pairs perfectly with the crunchy greens. And the savory granola, which I hope you always keep a jar of after this, provides crunch like a crouton and is filled with some of my favorite pantry items, like pumpkin seeds, oats, and puffed quinoa. The recipe calls for garlic powder instead of garlic cloves so that the granola can get nice and crunchy without any worry that the garlic will burn. Finally, the little gem. Sure, you could use another green for this, but why would you want to? Little gem has the perfect amount of nooks to scoop up all the delicious toppings, which is a must. **SERVES 4 TO 6**

2 small heads little gem lettuce

2 Persian cucumbers, thinly sliced

3 radishes, thinly sliced

1 shallot, thinly sliced

Savory Granola (recipe follows), for serving

FOR THE SHALLOT VINAIGRETTE

1 small shallot, finely chopped

1 tablespoon Dijon mustard

¼ cup extra virgin olive oil

Juice of 1 lemon (about 3 tablespoons)

¼ teaspoon fine sea salt

¼ teaspoon freshly ground black pepper

1 tablespoon rice vinegar

2 tablespoons nutritional yeast

1. Cut the ends off the little gem lettuce. Combine the lettuce, cucumbers, radishes, and sliced shallot together in a large bowl, reserving some veggies for garnish.

2. MAKE THE VINAIGRETTE: In a small bowl, whisk together the shallots, mustard, olive oil, lemon juice, salt, pepper, rice vinegar, and nutritional yeast until smooth.

3. Pour the dressing over the salad and toss to combine. To serve, garnish with the reserved veggies. Top with savory granola.

(continued)

savory granola

MAKES 3 CUPS

1½ cups organic rolled oats

½ cup pumpkin seeds

½ cup sliced almonds

½ cup puffed quinoa

2 tablespoons sesame seeds

2 egg whites

⅓ cup extra virgin olive oil

1 tablespoon garlic powder

1 teaspoon fine sea salt

1 teaspoon dried oregano

¼ teaspoon freshly ground black pepper

1. Preheat the oven to 350°F and line a baking sheet with parchment paper.

2. Combine the oats, pumpkin seeds, sliced almonds, puffed quinoa, and sesame seeds in a large bowl.

3. In a small bowl, whisk together the egg whites, olive oil, garlic powder, salt, oregano, and pepper. Pour the wet ingredients into the dry ingredients and mix until the dry ingredients are completely coated.

4. Spread the mixture on the baking sheet and flatten with a spatula.

5. Bake for 30 minutes. Stir the granola around with the spatula and bake for an additional 15 minutes, until the granola is golden brown and toasted.

6. Let the granola cool completely before storing in an airtight container at room temperature. It should stay good for about 3 weeks.

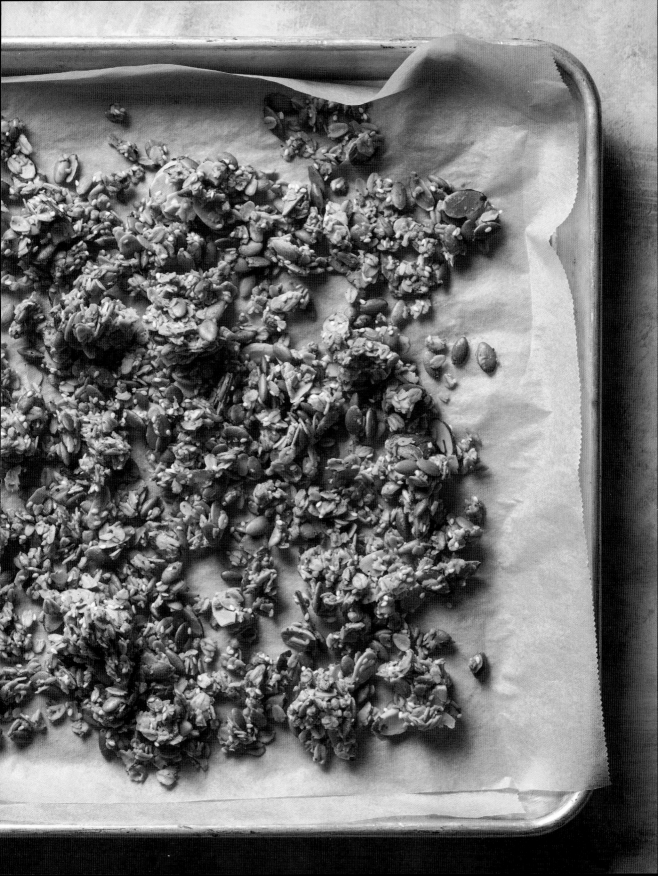

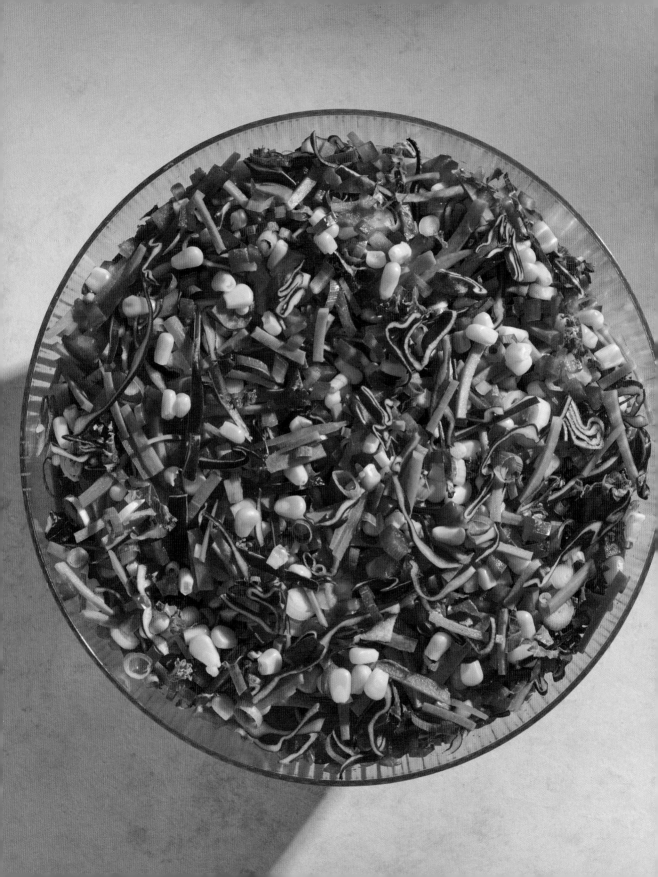

rainbow kale salad

When Adi and I first moved in together, we loved cooking for our friends and family every Sunday. They would come over and hang out as we cooked, dipping chips into the salads that were ready while we finished up the rest of the meal.

On those Sundays, I'd often make a variation of this salad, using all the bright, rainbow-colored veggies I loved most. You can use any vegetable or colors you want in this salad (it's hard to go wrong when there's such a delicious dressing), just remember to cut everything into the same size. I season the crunchy chickpeas with za'atar, a Middle Eastern spice blend of oregano, thyme, marjoram, sumac, and toasted sesame seeds. There are endless variations of za'atar blends depending on where you buy it (we normally get ours at the shuk in Israel), but they all add incredible brightness and flavor to whatever you use them on. **SERVES 6 TO 8**

1 bunch kale (about ½ pound), stems removed, leaves sliced into thin ribbons (see page 251)

2 or 3 red bell peppers, thinly sliced and cut into ½-inch pieces

2 or 3 carrots, finely chopped into ½-inch pieces

One 15-ounce can yellow corn, drained

1 head red cabbage, shredded and cut into small ½-inch pieces

1 bunch scallions, trimmed, white and light green parts cut into ¼-inch slices

Crunchy Za'atar Chickpeas (recipe follows), for serving

Grilled Soy Tofu (recipe follows), for serving

FOR THE MISO VINAIGRETTE

⅓ cup extra virgin olive oil

Juice of 2 lemons (about ⅓ cup)

¼ cup red wine vinegar

¼ cup white miso paste

⅓ cup nutritional yeast

1 tablespoon dried oregano

2 garlic cloves, grated with a Microplane

½ teaspoon fine sea salt

1. Make a bed with the kale ribbons. Arrange the bell pepper, carrots, corn, red cabbage, and scallions in a rainbow wheel on top.

2. MAKE THE VINAIGRETTE: Whisk together the olive oil, lemon juice, vinegar, miso paste, nutritional yeast, oregano, garlic, and salt in a bowl or jar until combined.

3. Pour the vinaigrette over the salad. Top with crunchy za'atar chickpeas and grilled soy tofu.

(continued)

crunchy za'atar chickpeas

MAKES 1 CUP

1 cup chickpeas, drained and rinsed

3 tablespoons extra virgin olive oil

1 teaspoon za'atar

1 teaspoon fine sea salt

2 garlic cloves, grated with a Microplane

1. Preheat the oven to 420°F and line a large baking sheet with parchment paper.

2. Dry the chickpeas well and add to a medium bowl with the olive oil, za'atar, salt, and garlic. Stir to combine.

3. Spread the chickpeas evenly on the baking sheet and roast for 20 to 30 minutes, stirring about halfway through, until crispy.

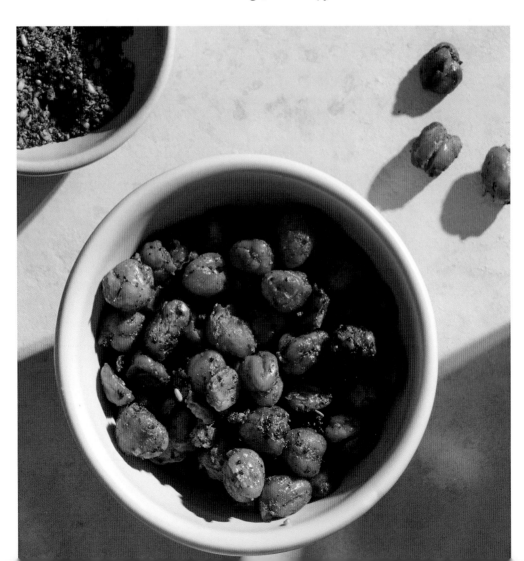

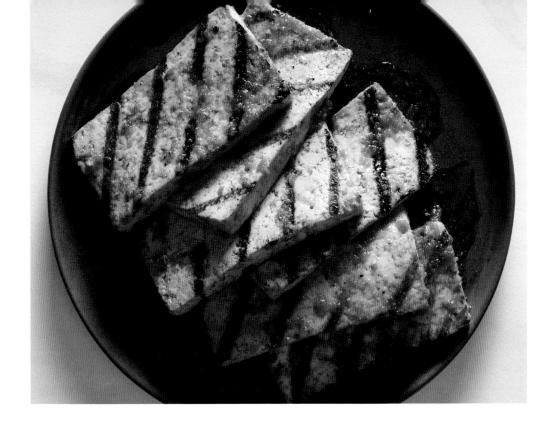

grilled soy tofu
You can use either a grill or a grill pan to get caramelized grill marks on both sides. **SERVES 4**

1 block extra-firm tofu

¼ cup avocado oil

2 tablespoons toasted sesame oil

2 tablespoons regular soy sauce

2 garlic cloves, grated with a Microplane

Juice of ½ lemon (about 1½ tablespoons)

1 tablespoon garlic powder

¼ teaspoon fine sea salt

1 teaspoon honey

1. Slice the tofu into ¾-inch rectangular slices.

2. Lay the sliced tofu flat on a kitchen towel and press the moisture out with another towel. Lay the tofu on a new dry towel to continue to pull moisture out.

3. Whisk together the oils, soy sauce, grated garlic, lemon juice, garlic powder, salt, and honey in a bowl to create the marinade.

4. Add the tofu to the marinade, cover, and place in the fridge for at least 20 minutes and up to 1 hour.

5. Heat a grill pan or grill over medium-high heat. Grill the marinated tofu to get nice grill marks, about 3 minutes on each side. Serve with your favorite salad to add extra protein.

the og iceberg

The very first time I went to Israel with Adi we landed in the afternoon. We had been dating for about a year and I had never met his family, so I was filled with nerves. I had been to Israel a few times as a kid, but I never could have imagined I would return someday with my boyfriend/future husband for Passover. It had been three years since Adi had left home with a backpack for a two-week trip to the United States; needless to say, his parents were so excited to see him.

His dad picked us up at the train station and drove us back to their house, where his mom had dinner waiting. We sat down and she put a big bowl of this very salad right in front of me. I was intrigued—it looked like lightly dressed iceberg. But I tried it, and my mind was blown. It will forever be my mother-in-law's salad, because she's the only person who has ever made it for me. I knew from that one bite that I wanted it to be in my life forever, just like her son. It's simple, requiring only six ingredients to make the vinaigrette, but it's so refreshing and satisfying at the same time. Just remember to dress it right before you eat so the iceberg stays crisp. **SERVES 4 TO 6**

1 head iceberg lettuce, chopped as desired (I prefer small bites)

Juice of 2 lemons (about ⅓ cup)

3 tablespoons extra virgin olive oil

1½ tablespoons white vinegar, or a healthy splash

2 large garlic cloves, finely chopped

¾ teaspoon fine sea salt

¼ teaspoon freshly ground black pepper

1. Place the iceberg in a large bowl.

2. Whisk together the lemon juice, olive oil, vinegar, garlic, salt, and pepper in a bowl or jar until combined.

3. Pour the dressing over the lettuce just before serving and toss to make sure everything is evenly coated. Serve immediately.

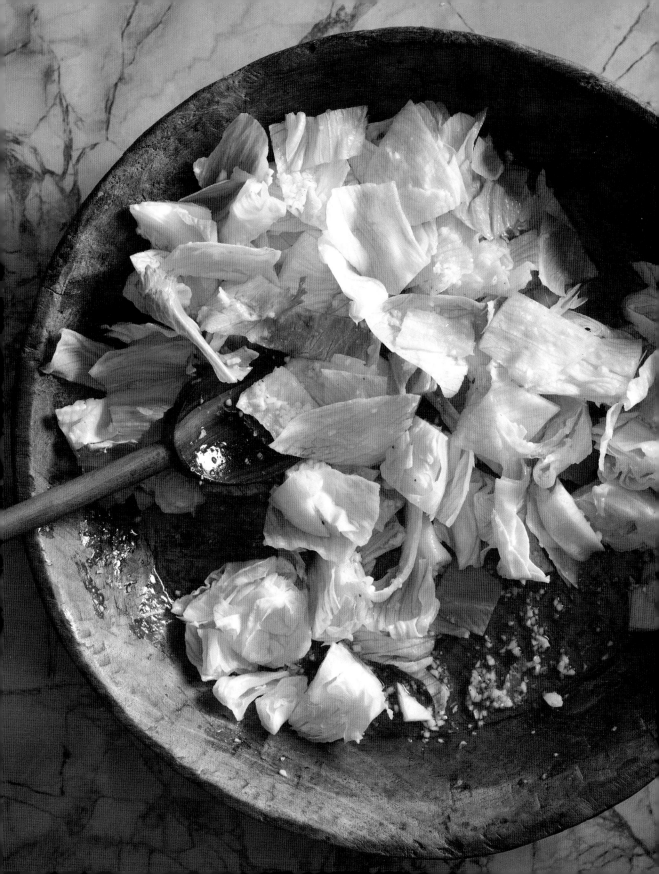

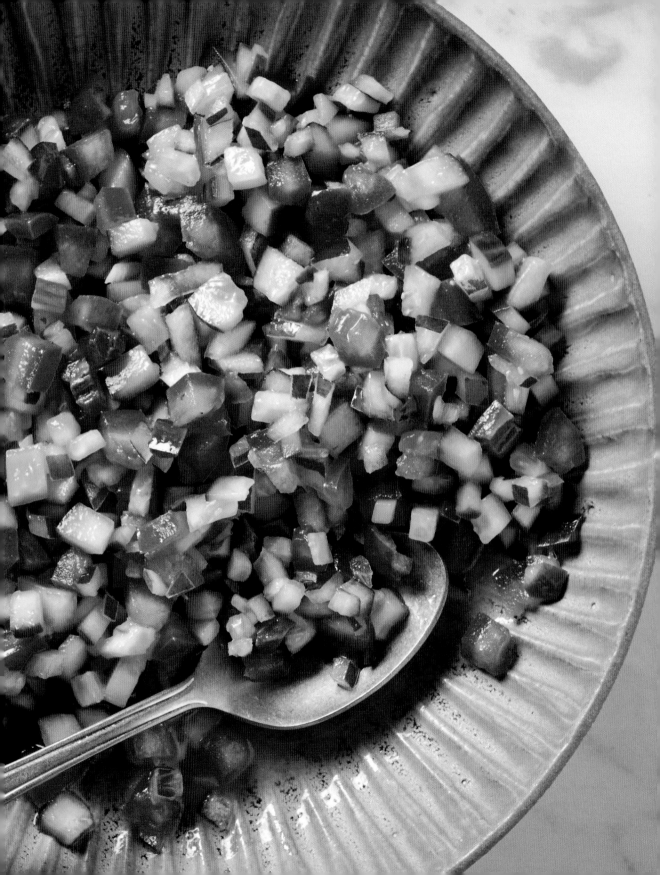

mediterranean chopped salad

This salad is the reason I married my husband. Well, sort of. On that same trip to Israel when I met Adi's parents, his mom made this salad with fresh, colorful produce. It was better than delicious—it was an inspiration.

Something I've learned as I get older and meet new people is that so many cultures have similar dishes with slight differences depending on where they're made, this one included. In Iran, you'll find mint added to the veggies in the similar salad-e Shirazi; in Syria, Lebanon, and Palestine, fattoush salads often include pomegranate and crunchy pita. Since Israel is a newer country, this salad was absolutely inspired by dishes of surrounding countries. Isn't it beautiful to think of food as what brings us together rather than what tears us apart?

I encourage you to think of this salad as a blank canvas and make it your own—I keep it light on onion and add Kalamata olives for a salty bite. Go ahead, play around with different herbs and vegetables you have on hand. It's so simple, so delicious, and is absolutely near and dear to my heart. **SERVES 4 TO 6**

6 to 8 Persian cucumbers (or 2 large cucumbers, seeds removed), cut into confetti-size pieces

4 Roma tomatoes, cut into confetti-size pieces

1 small red onion, cut into confetti-size pieces

¼ cup pitted Kalamata olives, finely chopped

FOR THE DRESSING

Juice of 2 lemons (about ⅓ cup)

¼ cup extra virgin olive oil

1 teaspoon fine sea salt

1. Combine the cucumbers, tomatoes, onion, and olives in a large bowl.

2. MAKE THE DRESSING: Add the lemon juice, olive oil, and salt to the bowl and stir to combine. Adjust seasonings to taste.

3. Store any leftovers in the fridge in an airtight container for 3 to 5 days. Use them to make the Mediterranean Toast (page 52).

green goddess salad

Like most goddesses, this salad needs no introduction. She's creamy, tangy, and filled with delicious green nutrients. Finely chopping all the vegetables is the most time-consuming part of making this salad, since the dressing comes together quickly in the blender. The best part is how versatile the recipe is. You can use lime instead of lemon, add a jalapeño or avocado, and mix and match the base veggies to create the salad of your dreams. Use leftovers to make the Green Goddess Toast (page 56), serve with tacos, or keep dipping your chips in it. **SERVES 10**

1 small head green cabbage, sliced into 1-inch ribbons, then cut into confetti-size pieces

3 to 4 Persian cucumbers (or 1 large cucumber with seeds removed), cut into confetti-size pieces

¼ cup fresh chives, chopped

1 bunch scallions, trimmed, white and light green parts cut into ¼-inch slices

FOR THE DRESSING

¼ cup extra virgin olive oil

Juice of 2 lemons (about ⅓ cup)

2 tablespoons rice vinegar

1 cup packed fresh basil leaves

1 cup fresh spinach

2 garlic cloves

1 small shallot

¼ cup nuts of your choice (I use raw, unsalted cashews)

⅓ cup nutritional yeast

1 teaspoon fine sea salt

Handful of fresh chives (optional)

1. Combine the cabbage, cucumbers, chives, and scallions in a large bowl.

2. MAKE THE DRESSING: Add the olive oil, lemon juice, and rice vinegar to a large high-powered blender. Cover with the basil, spinach, garlic, shallot, nuts, nutritional yeast, salt, and chives, if using, and blend until the dressing is smooth and creamy.

3. Pour the dressing over the salad and mix well.

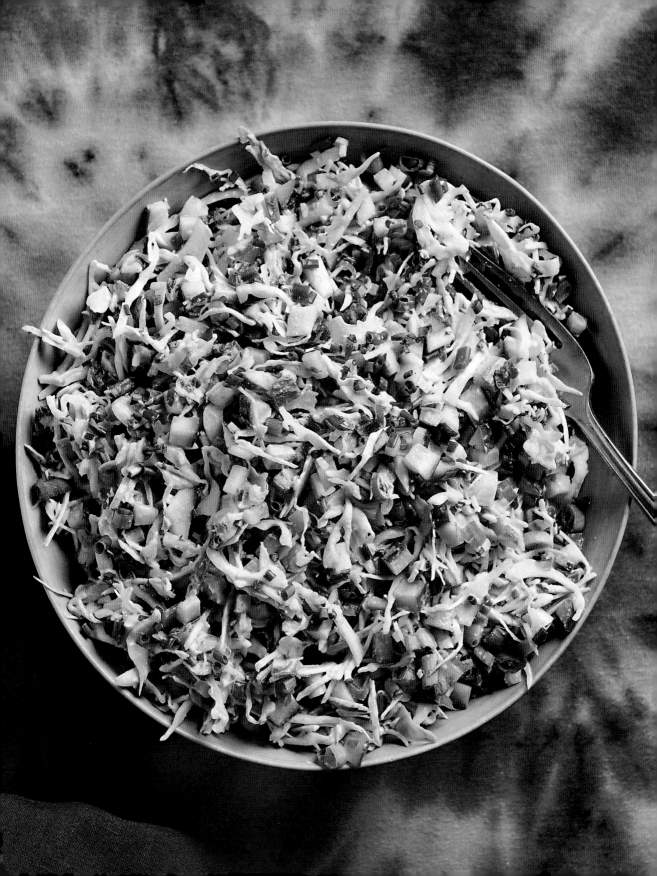

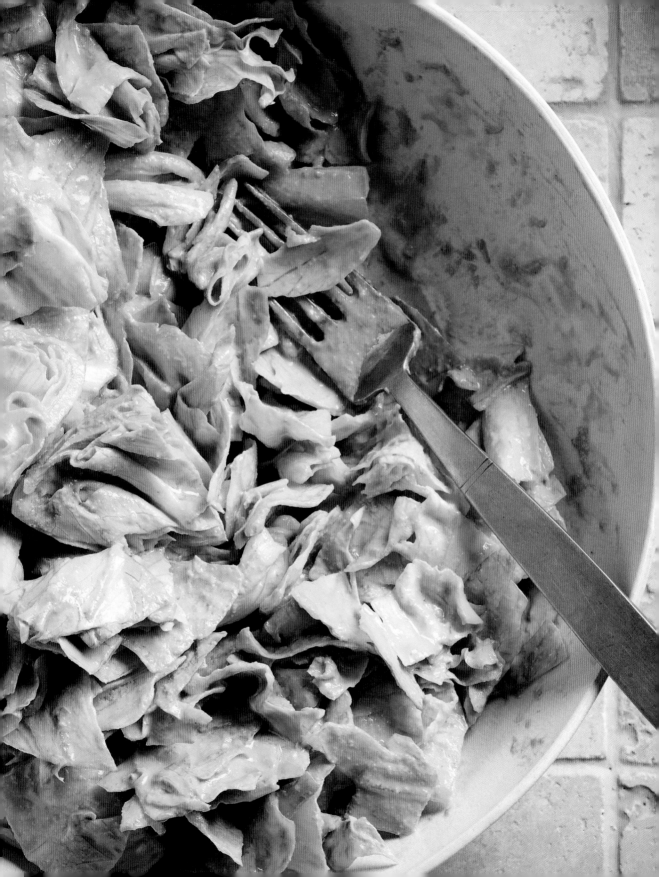

green goddess ranch salad

Imagine the Green Goddess had a younger, tangier sister. She'd be the Green Goddess Ranch, aka Mother Nature's Ranch. She's nothing like the bottled, milky, herby dressing I grew up on and loved to eat with chunks of cucumber, but she's packed with delicious nutrients. What makes it ranch-like are the dill and chives—two quintessential flavors of the classic dressing. Of course, you can't beat the bright-green hue from the spinach and herbs either. I like to serve this with iceberg for texture and crunch, but if you prefer you can use the OG Green Goddess base of cabbage and cucumbers (see page 98). **SERVES 6**

FOR THE DRESSING

⅓ cup extra virgin olive oil

Juice of 2 lemons (about ⅓ cup)

1 small shallot

2 to 3 garlic cloves

1 cup fresh spinach

1 cup fresh chives

1 cup fresh dill

¼ cup nutritional yeast

1 cup raw, unsalted cashews

1 scallion, trimmed

1 teaspoon fine sea salt

1 head iceberg lettuce

1. MAKE THE DRESSING: Add the olive oil and lemon juice to a large high-powered blender. Cover with the shallot, garlic, spinach, chives, dill, nutritional yeast, cashews, scallion, and salt and pulse until the dressing is smooth.

2. Chop the iceberg into small pieces and place in a large bowl.

3. Pour the dressing over the iceberg in the bowl and mix well to evenly coat. Serve immediately.

tahina cole slaw

One of our kitchen staples is tahini, or tahina, a paste made from ground sesame seeds. The paste adds a dairy-free, nutty creaminess to any dish you use it on, so we always have it on hand to dress up a meal. When I met Adi, I definitely called it "tahini," but over time he has influenced me in many ways, from how I eat to how I pronounce tahina (ta-KHEE-na, with a vibration in the back of the throat in the middle syllable). When you buy tahina at a store, it's pure sesame paste. To turn it into a pourable, flavorful condiment, I typically add water, lemon juice, and garlic to start, adding extra flavors or herbs depending on the recipe. The dressing is absolutely my favorite part of this salad because it pairs so well with the crunchy veggies and fresh herbs. Make sure to pay close attention to the size of the veggie chop here to make a truly stunning slaw. **SERVES 8 TO 10**

½ **head red cabbage or 1 small head red cabbage, thinly sliced into ribbons (I use a mandoline)**

1 red bell pepper, thinly sliced

3 carrots, peeled and grated or julienne-cut

1 bunch scallions, trimmed, light green and white parts cut into ¼-inch slices

½ **bunch fresh parsley, finely chopped**

FOR THE DRESSING

½ **cup tahina**

2 tablespoons Dijon mustard

2 garlic cloves, grated with a Microplane

1 teaspoon fine sea salt

¼ **teaspoon freshly ground black pepper**

Juice of 2 lemons (about ⅓ cup)

1 tablespoon rice vinegar

2 teaspoons honey

1. Combine the cabbage, bell pepper, carrots, scallions, and parsley in a bowl.

2. MAKE THE DRESSING: Whisk the tahina with ⅓ cup water in a medium bowl. It's going to get thick and separate, but then it will get thinner. Add more water until it reaches a mustard-like consistency.

3. Add the mustard, garlic, salt, black pepper, lemon juice, rice vinegar, and honey. Whisk to combine.

4. Coat the vegetables with the dressing, toss to evenly coat, and serve immediately.

tip: If you make this slaw in advance, keep the dressing separate so the slaw retains its crunch.

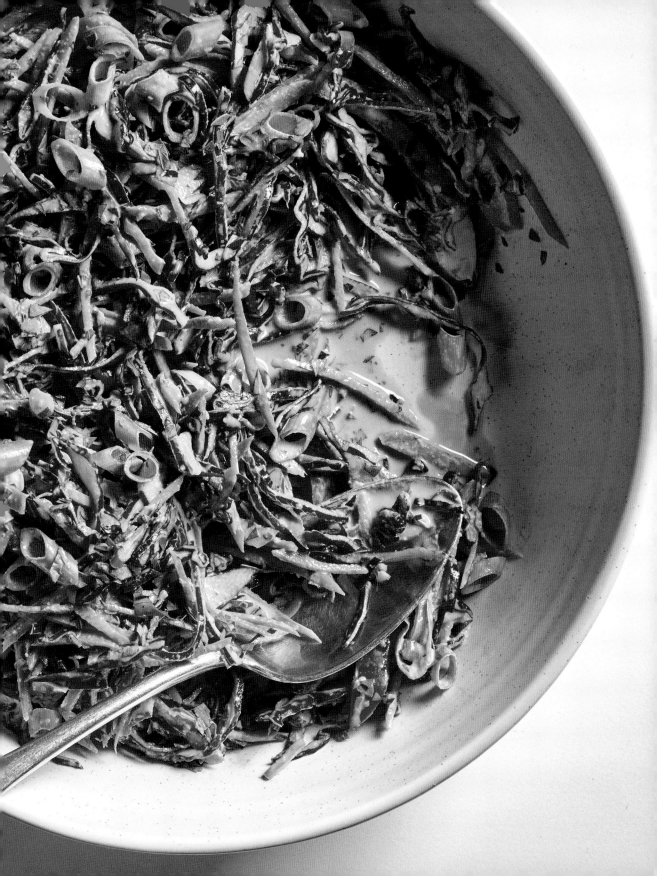

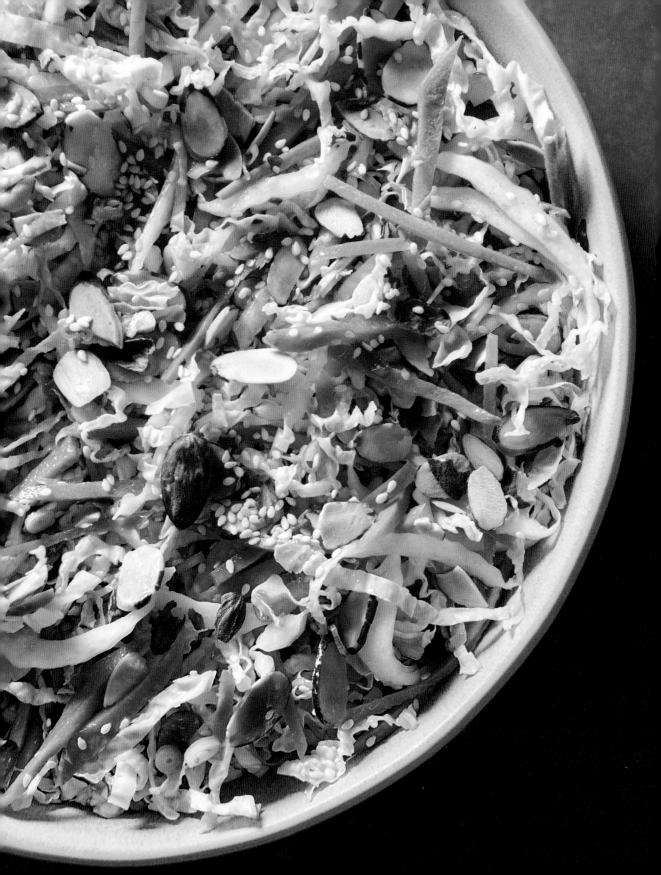

summer slaw

Some of my best inspiration for salads comes from the grocery store. I love to wander the aisles and see if there are any new ingredients I haven't seen before, but I really love a good salad bar. When I was in college, I could make the most delicious meals from even the humblest of salad bars. This recipe was inspired by a prepared salad at my local supermarket and relies wholly on proper ratios—the vegetables all add a unique crunch, and the sesame flavor comes through in the dressing and seeds. Cabbage heads tend to be huge, which is why I call for only half, but if you have a smaller one, go ahead and use the whole thing. The result is a refreshing, delicious salad that pairs perfectly with grilled chicken for added protein. **SERVES 4 TO 6**

1 cup sliced almonds

¼ cup sesame seeds

½ head savoy cabbage, finely shredded with a mandoline (about 3 cups)

4 medium carrots, peeled and grated

1 bunch scallions, trimmed, light green and white parts cut into ¼-inch slices

FOR THE DRESSING

3 tablespoons avocado oil

¼ cup toasted sesame oil

Juice of 1 lemon (about 3 tablespoons)

2 tablespoons white vinegar

1 heaping teaspoon honey

1 teaspoon fine sea salt

1. Place the almonds and sesame seeds together in a pan over medium heat until toasted, 3 to 5 minutes. Toss occasionally so they don't burn.

2. Combine the cabbage, carrots, and scallions in a large bowl.

3. Stir in most of the toasted almonds and sesame seeds, reserving some for garnish.

4. MAKE THE DRESSING: Whisk together the oils, lemon juice, vinegar, honey, and salt in a small bowl.

5. Pour the dressing over the salad and toss to combine. Garnish with the remaining almonds and sesame seeds. Serve immediately. If you make this in advance, store the dressing and salad separately in airtight containers in the fridge until you're ready to serve.

farm stand salad

Consider this salad my love letter to the farmers' market, where the produce is covered in dirt and tastes so much better than vegetables you buy at the grocery store. Garlic scapes—the green, curled stems that grow out of a garlic bulb—and scallions give a sharp bite, corn lends a hint of sweetness, snap peas offer crunch, and tomatoes burst with juices. If you can't find garlic scapes, just add extra scallions. By pouring the hot corn over all the aromatics, the herb and garlic flavors bloom and prove just how good a farm-fresh haul can be. **SERVES 8 TO 10**

2 tablespoons plus 1 teaspoon fine sea salt

4 corn cobs, shucked

1 bunch garlic scapes, finely chopped (optional)

4 red scallions, trimmed, light purple and white parts cut into ¼-inch slices

1 stalk young garlic, chopped

¼ cup roughly chopped fresh cilantro or parsley, plus more for garnish

Juice of 2 lemons (about ⅓ cup)

¼ cup extra virgin olive oil

¼ teaspoon freshly ground black pepper

1 cup snap peas, trimmed and cut on a bias

1 cup cherry tomatoes, cut in half

1 orange bell pepper, finely chopped

2 medium carrots, julienned

4 or 5 pink radishes, cut into small matchsticks

½ cup crumbled feta

1. Fill a large pot with cold water and add 2 tablespoons of the salt. Turn the heat up to medium-high/high and add the corn. Once the water reaches a rapid boil, take the pot off the heat and cover until you're ready to use the corn. (It won't overcook, I promise.)

2. Add the scapes, if using, scallions, garlic, and cilantro—the aromatics—to a large bowl. Cover with the lemon juice, the remaining 1 teaspoon salt, the olive oil, and black pepper and whisk to combine. If it smells amazing, you're doing it right.

3. Carefully cut the corn kernels off the cob while still hot. To safely get the kernels off, start by cutting the ends off the cob so it can stand up easily. Place the cob vertically in a large bowl (which will help catch any flying kernels) and anchor it with a corn holder or fork. Then use a sharp knife to cut the kernels off, being careful not to cut too closely since the end is hard and fibrous. Add the kernels to the bowl with the aromatics. The warmth from the corn helps the flavor of the aromatics bloom.

4. Add the snap peas, tomatoes, bell pepper, and radishes to the bowl. Stir to combine so everything is evenly coated with the dressing. Garnish with more cilantro and the feta.

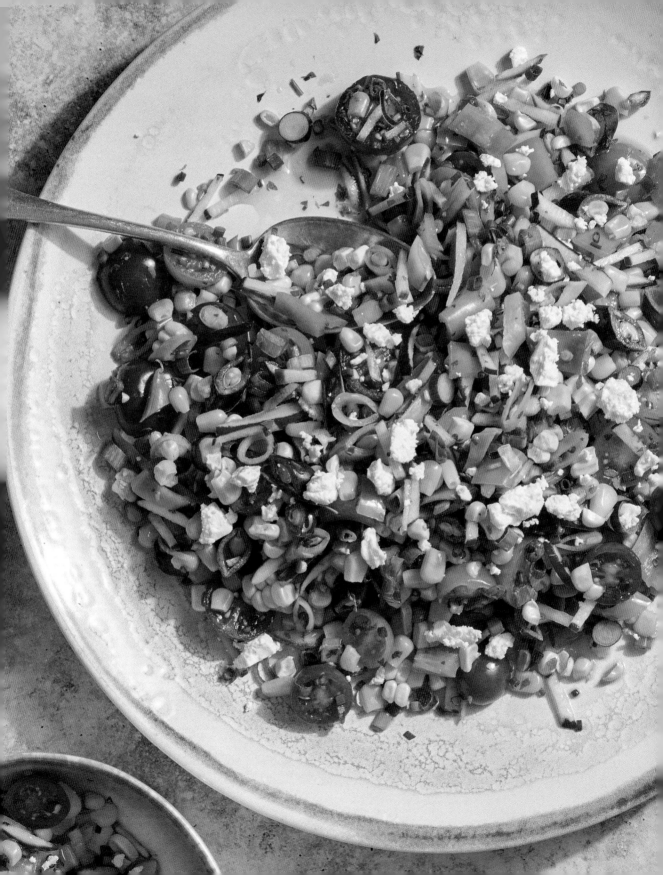

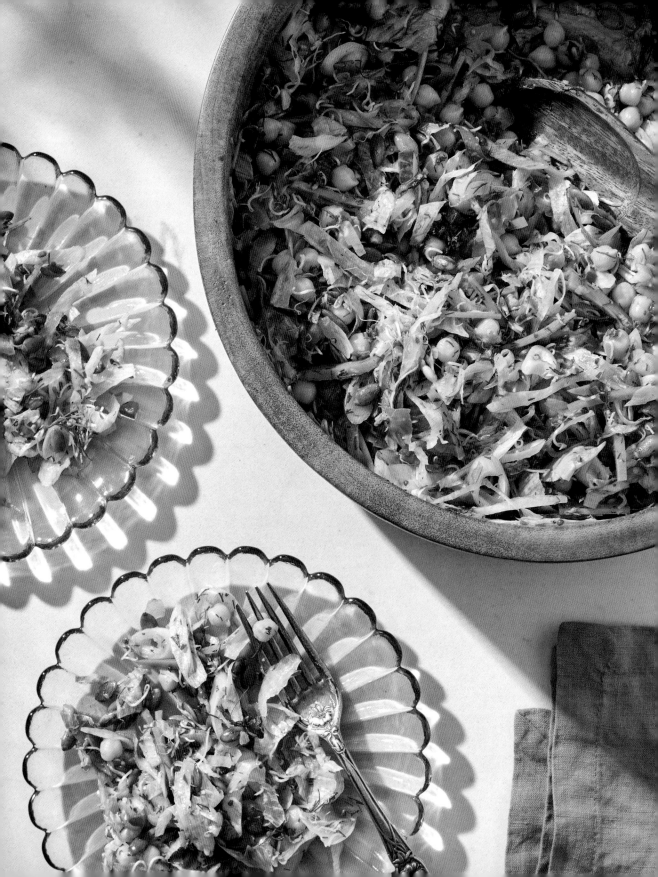

sprouted salad

I consider sprouts a superfood—they're packed with powerful antioxidants and grow easily in less than a week. They're essentially young plants, which means they're one of the most nutrient-dense ingredients on the planet. As an aspiring gardener, I discovered how easy it is to grow sprouts myself, which was a game changer for my salads. Sprouting doesn't require a lot of space, sunlight, or expensive tools (see my how-to on page 266), and it saves so much money over time. I love knowing exactly where my vegetables are coming from, and this salad deliciously showcases my homegrown creations. **SERVES 4 TO 6**

1 head romaine lettuce, cut into ¼-inch pieces

1 red bell pepper, thinly sliced and cut into 1-inch pieces

2 medium carrots, julienned

1 bunch scallions, trimmed, light green and white parts cut into ¼-inch slices

One 15-ounce can chickpeas, drained and rinsed

1 cup sprouts, chopped (any mix of your choice—I use sprouted lentils, sprouted mung beans, alfalfa sprouts, and broccoli sprouts)

FOR THE DRESSING

¼ cup extra virgin olive oil

1 tablespoon Dijon mustard

1 garlic clove, minced

1 teaspoon honey

Juice of 2 lemons (about ⅓ cup)

½ teaspoon fine sea salt

½ teaspoon freshly ground black pepper

2 tablespoons nutritional yeast

Splash of rice vinegar

1. In a large bowl, toss together the romaine, bell pepper, carrots, scallions, chickpeas, and sprouts.

2. MAKE THE DRESSING: Whisk together the olive oil, mustard, garlic, honey, lemon juice, salt, black pepper, nutritional yeast, and rice vinegar in a small bowl.

3. Pour the dressing over the salad and mix to combine. Serve immediately.

beets & seeds

Sweet, crunchy, earthy, and hot pink—a few of my favorite things all in one bite. The best part of this salad is that it requires just enough preparation to make you feel like you made something truly spectacular, but not enough to overwhelm. Since it's served cold, it makes the perfect summer side or can be enjoyed as leftovers later. I think it tastes even better after a few days, when the beets soak up all the juices. Don't wear your favorite white shirt when you make this salad because the beet juice tends to get everywhere, but trust me, it's worth it! **SERVES 4 TO 6**

2 beets, trimmed

½ cup pumpkin seeds

Juice of 2 lemons (about ⅓ cup)

¼ cup extra virgin olive oil

2 tablespoons chopped garlic scapes, if you have them (leave out if it's not scape season)

2 garlic cloves, grated with a Microplane

2 tablespoons chopped fresh chives

½ teaspoon fine sea salt

¼ teaspoon freshly ground black pepper

½ cup crumbled feta

1. Wash and peel the beets. Grate the beets with a box grater or a food processor and place them in a large bowl.

2. Heat a large skillet over medium heat and add the pumpkin seeds. Cook until they start to smell nutty and turn golden brown, 5 to 7 minutes. Stir occasionally so they don't burn.

3. Add the lemon juice, olive oil, scapes, if using, the garlic, chives, salt, and pepper to the bowl with the beets. Toss until fully combined.

4. Top with the toasted pumpkin seeds and feta. Store leftovers in an airtight container in the fridge for 3 to 5 days. I like to eat my leftovers with cottage cheese!

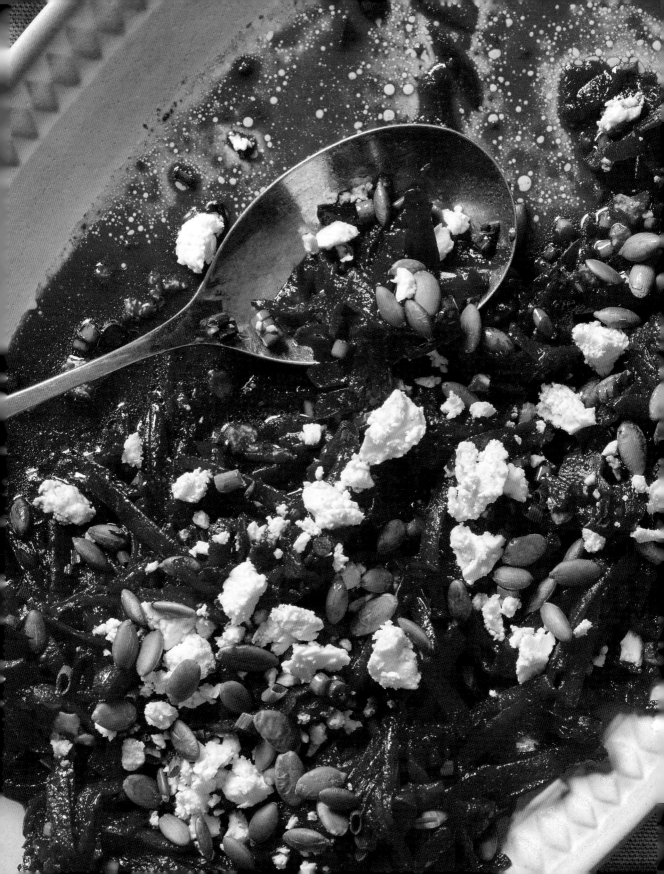

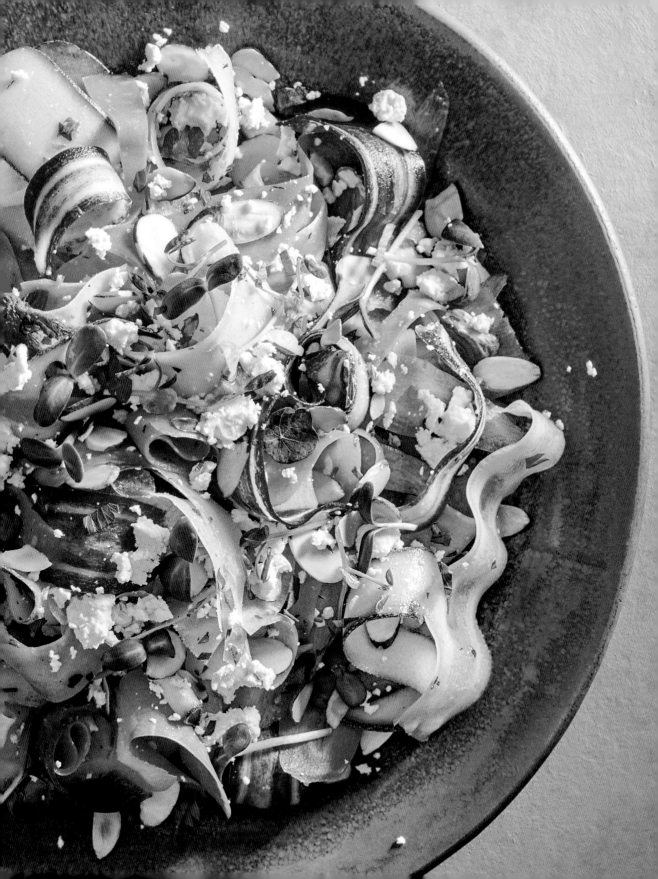

shaved carrot & zucchini salad

I'm not a fancy person—casual and laid-back has always been more my vibe. But let's face it, every now and then, it feels great to get all dressed up and go to a party. This salad is like that special event. It's perfect for those special times when you want to showcase gorgeous produce from the farmers' market and want your vegetables to twirl around your fork with the same ease as a long strip of pappardelle. It's a delicious, easy way to impress your guests and their taste buds. **SERVES 4 TO 6**

4 medium multicolored carrots, peeled

1 medium zucchini

1½ tablespoons finely chopped fresh parsley

1½ tablespoons finely chopped fresh cilantro

Juice of 1 lemon (about 3 tablespoons)

3 tablespoons extra virgin olive oil

½ teaspoon fine sea salt

¼ teaspoon freshly ground black pepper

½ teaspoon garlic powder

½ cup sliced almonds

½ cup crumbled feta

½ cup microgreens

1. Shave the carrots into ribbons with a Y peeler, which allows you to hold the vegetable in one hand and peel long strips with the other.

2. Shave the zucchini into similar ribbons, stopping when you reach the seeds and rotating the zucchini to get as many ribbons as you can.

3. Mix the ribbons together in a large bowl.

4. Whisk together the parsley, cilantro, lemon juice, olive oil, salt, pepper, and garlic powder in a small bowl.

5. Toss the salad together with the dressing and plate carefully. Garnish with the sliced almonds, feta, and microgreens. Store any leftovers in an airtight container in the fridge for 3 to 5 days.

edamame salad

My youngest daughter's favorite snack is edamame, so I always make sure we have a package of frozen edamame at the house. That very bag inspired this recipe, since it's so easy to make all of it—dressing included!—quickly in a pan. By adding the cabbage right when you turn off the flame, it keeps its crunch but warms slightly, mixing with the edamame for a gorgeous salad. My daughter hasn't yet graduated to this salad, but she'll get there. **SERVES 2 TO 3**

2 tablespoons toasted sesame oil

3 large garlic cloves, grated with a Microplane

2 tablespoons sesame seeds, plus more for garnish

One 12-ounce bag frozen shelled edamame

1 lemon, halved

½ teaspoon fine sea salt

½ head red cabbage, shredded and cut into 1-inch pieces

1. Start with a cold pan. Pour the oil into the pan and add the garlic and sesame seeds.

2. Turn the heat to medium-low and cook just until the garlic sizzles, about 3 to 5 minutes. Stir occasionally to infuse the oil with garlic, but don't let the garlic burn.

3. Add the edamame to the pan and cover. Let sit for 4 to 5 minutes to thaw the edamame. Remove the cover from the pan, increase the heat to medium, and let cook until the edamame starts to sizzle, about 5 minutes.

4. Take the pan off the heat and juice the lemon directly into the pan. Season with the salt and stir in the cabbage.

5. Transfer the salad to a large serving bowl. Garnish with sesame seeds and serve. Store any leftovers in an airtight container in the fridge for 3 to 5 days.

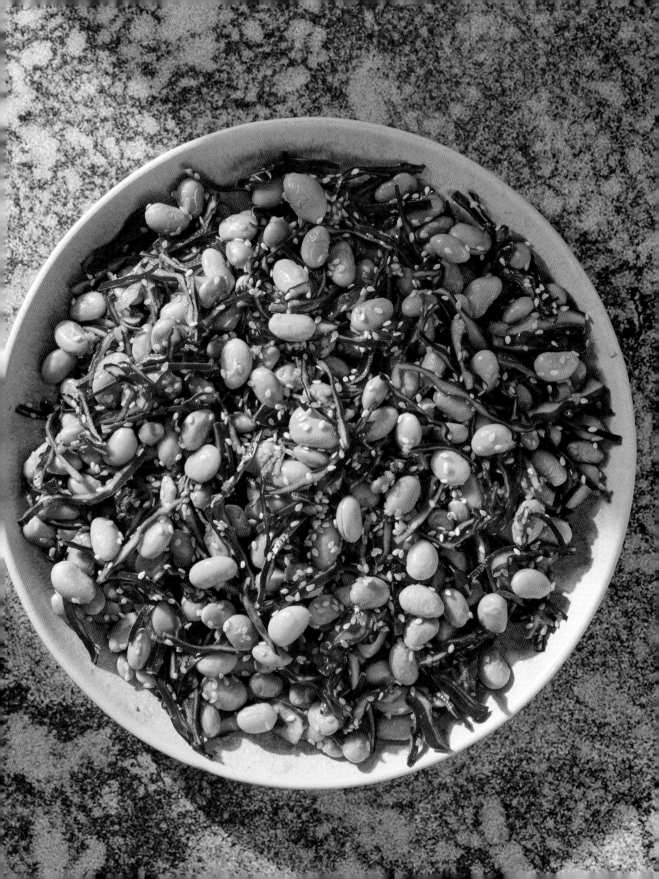

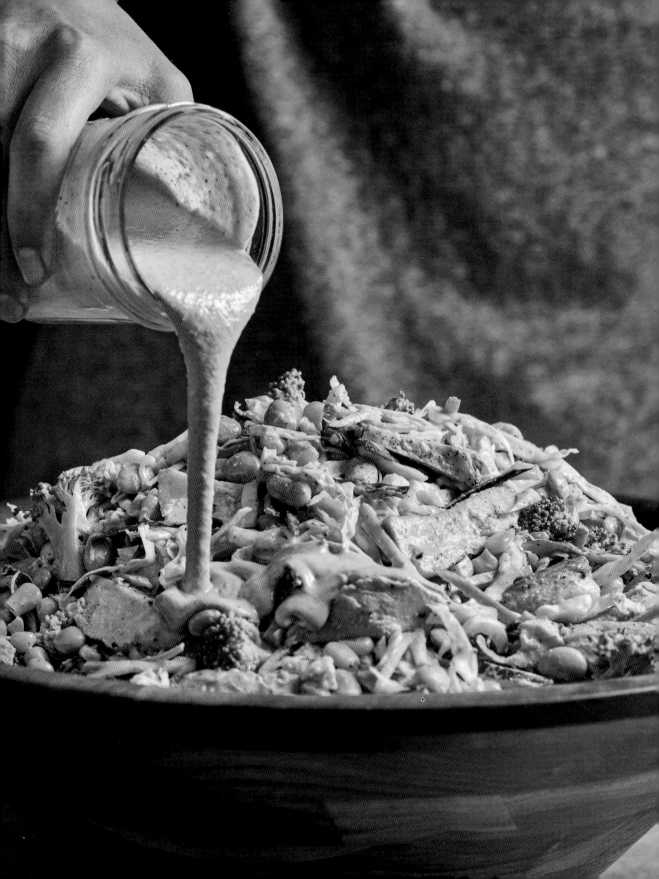

supermarket slaw

Next time you're going to a party and need to bring something, bring this. It's more over-the-top than your basic slaw, with different ingredients, a combination of raw and cooked vegetables, and a burst of bright flavor. All you have to do is go to the supermarket and get the prechopped bags of slaw and some frozen veggies, and this showstopping salad comes together in minutes. I love that the almonds give it a crunch and the feta lends the perfect amount of saltiness. I like to sauté bacon or pancetta with the vegetables for extra flavor, but you can leave it out if you prefer. Just remember that this feeds a crowd! **SERVES 10 TO 12**

One 4-ounce package pancetta

1 pound chicken breast, cooked using the Simple Grilled Chicken recipe (page 84), chopped

One 16-ounce bag frozen broccoli

2 cups sliced almonds

One 16-ounce bag frozen corn

One 12-ounce bag frozen shelled edamame

1 tablespoon oregano

1 tablespoon garlic powder

1 teaspoon fine sea salt

½ teaspoon freshly ground black pepper

3 tablespoons extra virgin olive oil

Two 12-ounce bags cole slaw mix (if your store has multiple options of cole slaw mixes, get two different kinds just for fun)

1 cup crumbled feta, to garnish

FOR THE DRESSING

⅓ cup store-bought pesto

Juice of 2 lemons (about ⅓ cup)

½ cup sour cream

Fine sea salt and freshly ground black pepper

1. Heat a large skillet over medium heat (no need to add oil). Add the pancetta and cook until the fat begins to render, 4 to 5 minutes.

2. Add the chicken, broccoli, almonds, corn, and edamame to the pan. Add the oregano, garlic powder, salt, and pepper. Drizzle with the olive oil and cook until the veggies are tender and thawed completely, 10 to 15 minutes, depending on the size of your pan. Remove from the heat.

3. MAKE THE DRESSING: Whisk together the pesto, lemon juice, and sour cream in a small bowl. Season with salt and pepper.

4. Combine the cole slaw bags in a large bowl. Don't use any of the packaged dressing, if it's included.

5. Add the cooked veggies and chicken to the cole slaw. Just before serving, pour the creamy pesto dressing on top and toss well to fully combine. Top with the feta and serve immediately.

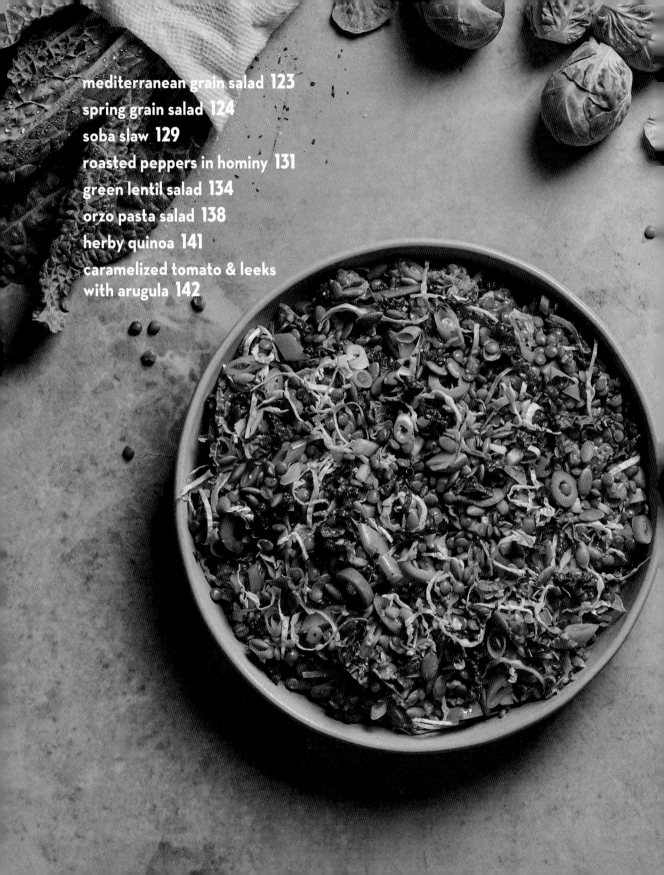

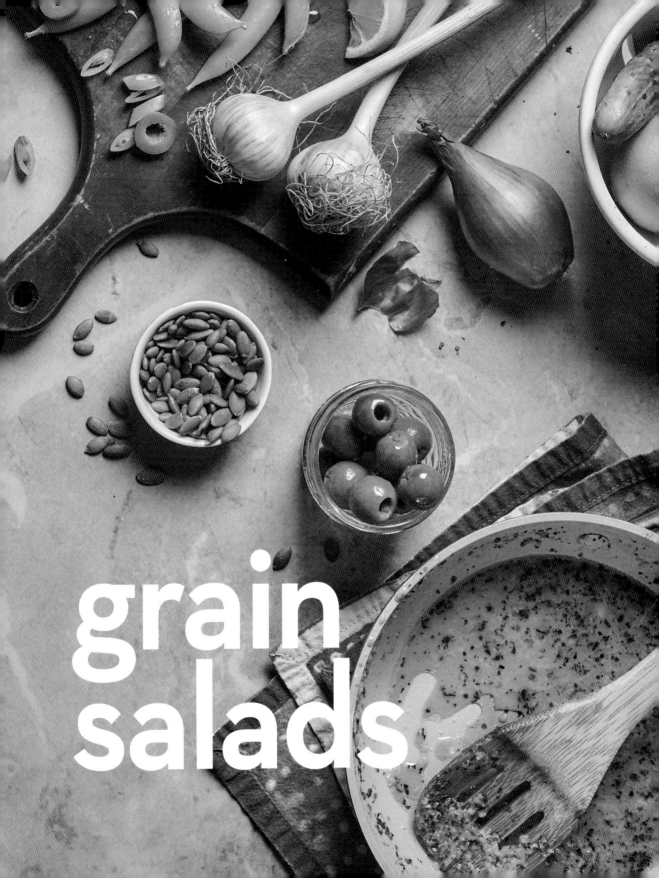

grain
salads

When I was little, my mom made a delicious pasta salad with Italian dressing, tomatoes, cucumbers, and broccoli. As my love for salads grew and I continued to experiment in the kitchen, this simple childhood staple has inspired so many different salads packed with hearty grains and lots of flavor.

At my house, I always have a variety of grains on hand. Farro, freekeh, rice, orzo, and even animal-shaped pasta help me make delicious, filling meals in a pinch while adding great texture and nutrients to meals. To make a truly mouthwatering grain salad, the best ratio of grains to greens is 1:1—try to think of grains as equal to the greens, with the veggies cut to match the size of the grain and portioned in equal ratios. And be generous with your dressings—they add incredible flavor and really bring the dish together. Included in this section are some of my go-to weeknight meals, because they come together quickly and have the perfect balance of greens and grains to end the day with food that makes me happy.

> **" My go-to weeknight meals have the perfect balance of greens and grains to end the day with food that makes me happy. "**

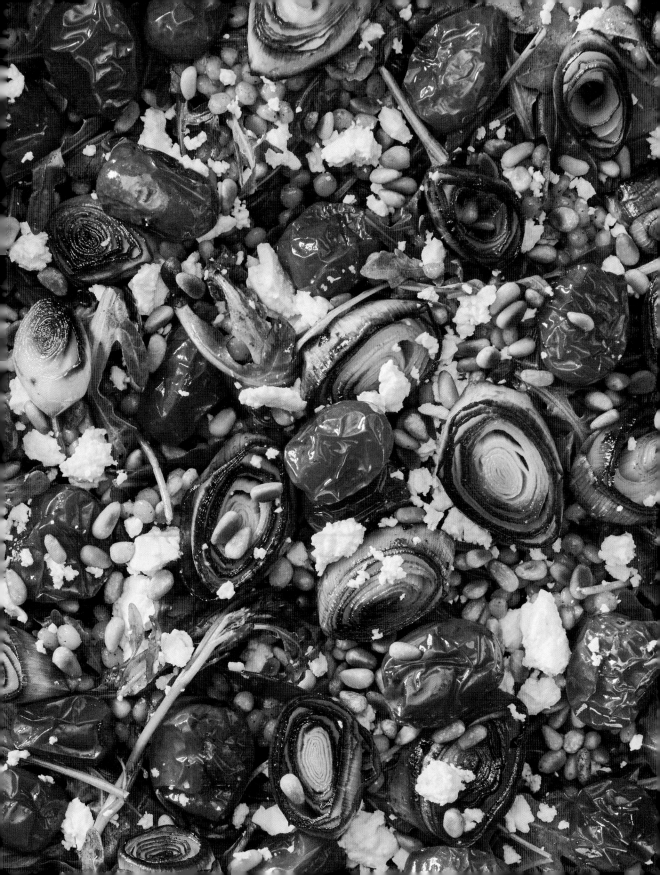

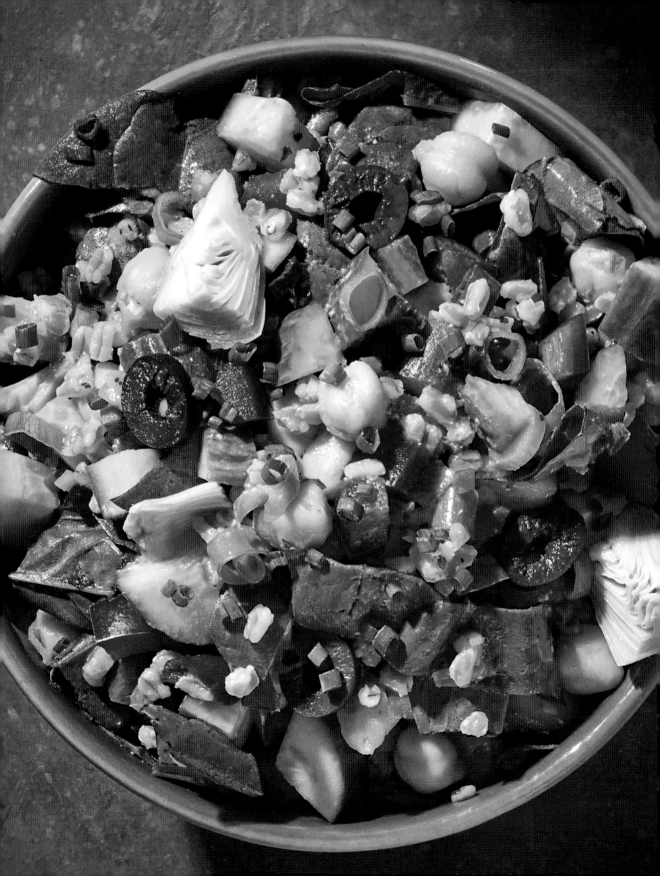

mediterranean grain salad

Grain salads offer endless opportunity. One night, I had leftover farro to use and only a few veggies in my fridge. I let the Mediterranean flavors I love inspire me and tossed the farro together with pantry staples (salty bites of olives, juicy artichoke hearts) and fresh spinach. The finely chopped raw veggies add just the right amount of crunch and flavor. My favorite part of this salad is that it really makes you feel good after you eat it, and it doesn't require intense planning. We now eat it on repeat on busy nights—I encourage you to do the same. **SERVES 4**

¼ teaspoon fine sea salt

½ cup uncooked farro

6 Persian cucumbers, cut into confetti-size pieces

1 cup fresh spinach, chopped

1 red bell pepper, finely chopped

One 15-ounce can chickpeas, drained and rinsed

Two 6.5-ounce jars artichoke hearts marinated in oil, chopped (I like the ones in glass jars because they are softer)

¼ cup pitted Kalamata olives, chopped

1 bunch scallions, trimmed, light green and white parts cut into ¼-inch slices

¼ cup chopped fresh chives

FOR THE DRESSING

¼ cup extra virgin olive oil

¼ cup red wine vinegar

1 garlic clove, grated with a Microplane

1 teaspoon dried oregano

2 tablespoons white miso paste

Juice of 1 lemon (about 3 tablespoons)

2 tablespoons nutritional yeast

1 teaspoon fine sea salt

1. Bring a medium pot with 1½ cups water to a boil. Once boiling, season the water with the salt and add the farro. Stir to combine and lower the heat so the water is simmering. Cook the farro, uncovered, until tender, about 30 minutes. Drain any excess water and let cool.

2. While the farro cooks, combine the cucumbers, spinach, bell pepper, chickpeas, artichokes, olives, scallions, and chives in a large bowl.

3. MAKE THE DRESSING: Whisk together the olive oil, vinegar, garlic, oregano, miso, lemon juice, nutritional yeast, and salt in a small bowl.

4. Add the cooled farro to the salad and stir to combine. Pour the dressing over the salad and mix to evenly coat. Store any leftovers in an airtight container in the fridge for 3 to 5 days.

spring grain salad

When you take your first bite of this bright, gorgeous salad, make sure you have a little of everything on your fork. This instruction applies to all my salads, but especially this one—it tastes just like springtime, promise. The recipe was inspired by the farmers' market in April, when I found myself buying the same things over and over and wanting to eat them all at once. The herby tahina adds a bright burst of flavor, and you can absolutely swap in your favorite herbs to create your perfect flavor profile. Just don't forget to add a generous drizzle of the dressing when you serve.

SERVES 6

½ teaspoon fine sea salt

1 cup uncooked farro

1 large bunch asparagus, about 1 inch of the ends cut off

1 cup snap peas, trimmed

1 bunch scallions, trimmed

6 radishes, trimmed

1 cup pumpkin seeds

FOR THE HERBY TAHINA VINAIGRETTE

1 cup tahina

Juice of 3 lemons (a bit more than ½ cup)

1½ tablespoons chopped fresh dill

¼ cup chopped fresh chives

2 garlic cloves, grated with a Microplane

1 teaspoon fine sea salt

1. Bring a medium pot with 3 cups water to a boil. Once boiling, season the water with the salt and add the farro. Stir to combine and lower the heat so the water is simmering. Cook the farro, uncovered, until tender, about 30 minutes. Drain any excess water and let cool.

2. Prepare an ice bath and have nearby. To blanch your veggies, bring a large pot of water to a boil and add the asparagus. Cook until the asparagus brightens in color and softens slightly, 3 to 4 minutes, then immediately transfer them to the ice bath for at least 1 minute to stop the cooking. Add the snap peas to the boiling water for 1½ minutes, then transfer to the ice bath.

3. Chop the asparagus into 1-inch pieces, the snap peas into ¼-inch pieces on a bias, the light green and white parts of the scallions into ¼-inch slices, and the radishes into thin slices.

4. Add the pumpkin seeds to a large dry skillet over medium heat. Don't leave these unattended! Every so often, pick up the pan and shake the seeds

(continued)

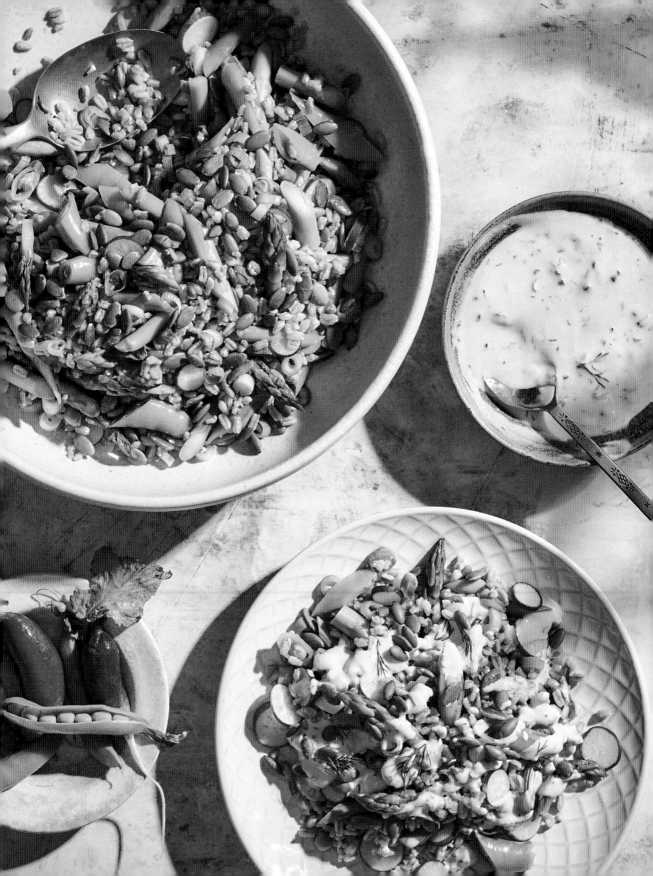

around so they don't burn. Remove the pan from the heat when the seeds begin to brown and have a nutty aroma, 5 to 7 minutes.

5. MAKE THE VINAIGRETTE: Whisk the tahina and lemon juice together with ¾ cup cold water in a small bowl, adding more water as needed until the mixture is smooth and pourable. It will get thick, then it will get thin again, but keep stirring until it reaches the right consistency. Add the herbs, garlic, and salt to the tahina and stir until mixed.

6. Combine the asparagus, snap peas, scallions, radishes, and farro in a large bowl. Drizzle with the herby tahina, garnish with toasted pumpkin seeds, and serve. Store any leftovers in an airtight container in the fridge for 3 to 5 days.

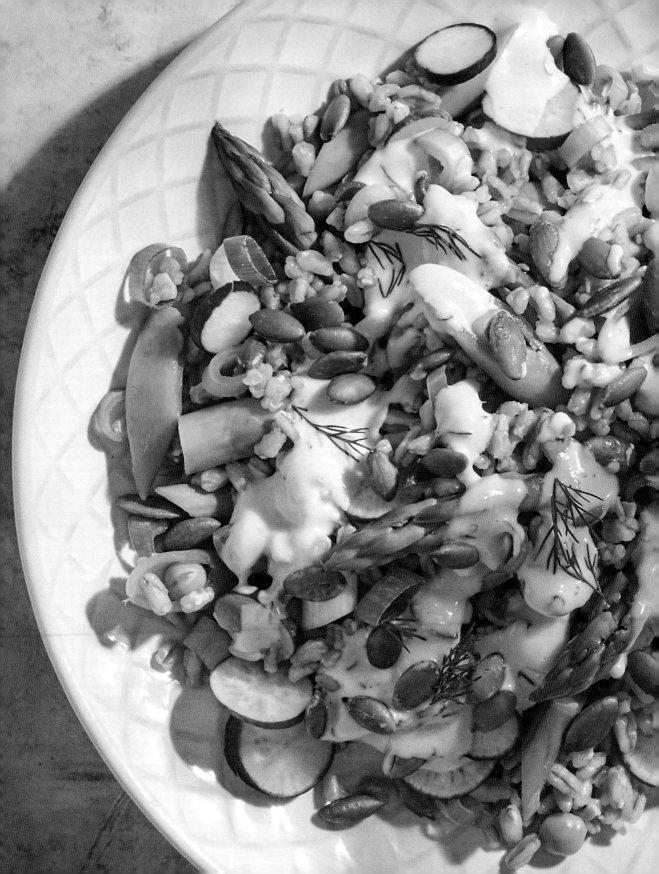

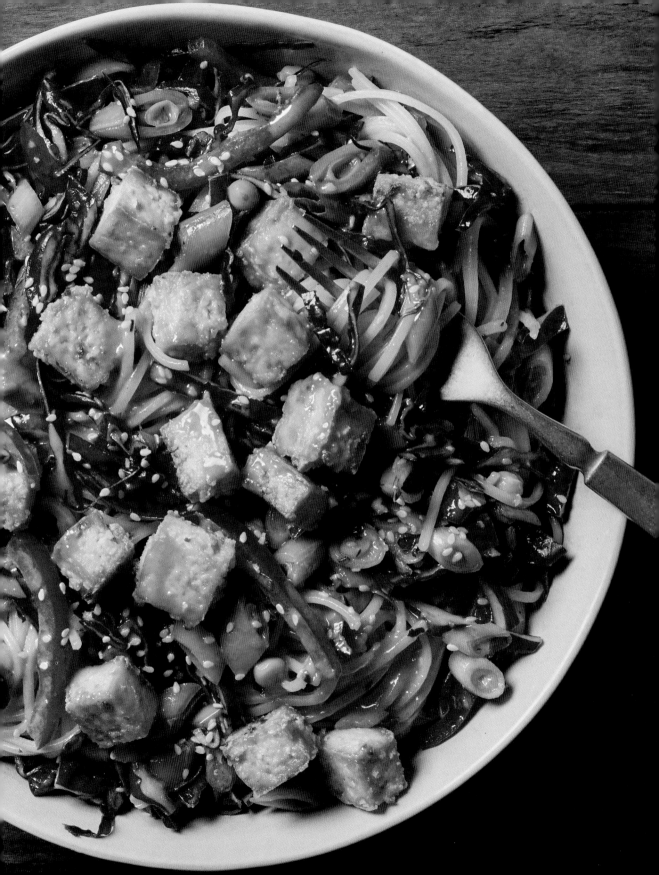

soba slaw One night, when I was fresh out of ideas, I asked Adi to tell me what to make for dinner. He began listing ingredients we had on hand, from fresh veggies to soba noodles. I started chopping. The results—coated in a silky soy-peanut dressing—were so good that this salad was added to our weekly meal rotation.

While this ended as a celebration of trying new things and using what you have, I think it also serves as a reminder to keep your pantry stocked with ingredients that excite you. Scour the aisles at your local grocery store for new pastas or grains so that you always have something interesting to throw together at a minute's notice. If you look in my pantry, you'll find a collection of various pastas; jars filled with grains; and an array of spices, with lemons, soy sauce, and vegetables like scallions, peppers, lettuces, and cucumbers filling the fridge. Frozen vegetables are also a staple in our house to create quick meals with lots of greens. **SERVES 4 TO 6**

½ **head red cabbage, shredded and cut into 1½-inch pieces**

½ **cup snap peas, trimmed and cut into ¼-inch pieces on a bias**

1 red bell pepper, thinly sliced and cut into 1½-inch pieces

1 bunch scallions, trimmed, white and light green parts cut into ¼-inch slices

2 tablespoons finely chopped fresh cilantro

Half of a 9.5-ounce package soba noodles, cooked according to package instructions and cooled

Crispy Tofu (recipe follows)

Sesame seeds, to garnish

FOR THE TOASTED SESAME SOY-PEANUT DRESSING

3 tablespoons regular soy sauce

3 tablespoons toasted sesame oil

1 tablespoon rice vinegar

Juice of 1 lemon (about 3 tablespoons)

1 tablespoon peanut butter

2 garlic cloves, grated with a Microplane

1. Mix together the cabbage, snap peas, bell pepper, scallions, and cilantro in a large bowl.

2. MAKE THE DRESSING: In a small bowl, whisk together the soy sauce, sesame oil, rice vinegar, lemon juice, peanut butter, and garlic until well combined. Pour the dressing over the vegetables and toss to get everything evenly coated.

3. Plate each dish individually by placing the soba noodles on the bottom, then covering with salad. Top with crispy tofu and garnish with sesame seeds.

note: For more of my pantry staples, see page 256.

(continued)

crispy tofu

SERVES 4

1 block extra-firm tofu

3 tablespoons avocado oil

4 garlic cloves, minced or grated with a Microplane

2 tablespoons cornstarch

1 teaspoon fine sea salt

¼ teaspoon freshly ground black pepper

1. Preheat the oven to 375°F and line a baking sheet with parchment paper.

2. Place the tofu on a tea towel and cut it into 1-inch cubes. Press out as much of the extra water as possible.

3. In a small bowl, whisk together the avocado oil and garlic.

4. Place the tofu in a large bowl and cover with the oil and garlic mixture. Sprinkle in the cornstarch and stir so the tofu is evenly coated. Season with salt and pepper.

5. Transfer the tofu to the baking sheet and bake for 25 minutes. Flip the tofu and bake for another 25 minutes, until crispy and golden.

roasted peppers in hominy

With the smokiness of roasted peppers, creamy feta, and the subtle sweetness of hominy, this salad is my homage to spicy Mexican elote. While the popular street corn features crumbly cotija cheese and a creamy chili sauce, this recipe adds smoky flavor to chewy, nutty hominy, which looks just like giant kernels of corn. The different colors of pepper don't matter in terms of taste, only for the color—a variety of colors helps create an eye-catching dish. Feel free to use more poblanos or jalapeños for a spicier dish and remember to soak the hominy overnight. Soaking makes it infinitely faster to cook the grain to the ideal al dente texture. **SERVES 6**

2 cups dried hominy

1 tablespoon fine sea salt

1 poblano pepper

2 bell peppers (one yellow and one red, for color)

1 jalapeño pepper

½ cup crumbled feta

1 tablespoon chopped fresh cilantro

1 tablespoon chopped fresh parsley

1. Add the dried hominy to a large heavy-bottomed saucepan and cover with filtered water. With the lid on, leave to soak for 8 hours or overnight (it's okay to let it sit at room temperature). Drain the hominy and return it to the saucepan. Cover with fresh water by about 2 inches. Add the salt and bring to a rapid boil over medium-high heat, then lower the heat to reduce it to a simmer. Cook the hominy for 2 hours, until it looks like a flower (kind of like a popped popcorn kernel).

2. Preheat the oven to broil and line a baking sheet with aluminum foil. Evenly place all the peppers on the sheet and broil until the tops are charred, 5 to 10 minutes. Flip the peppers and put them back under the broiler for another 5 minutes, or until the other side is charred.

3. Carefully place the peppers in a glass container and cover while the peppers cool.

(continued)

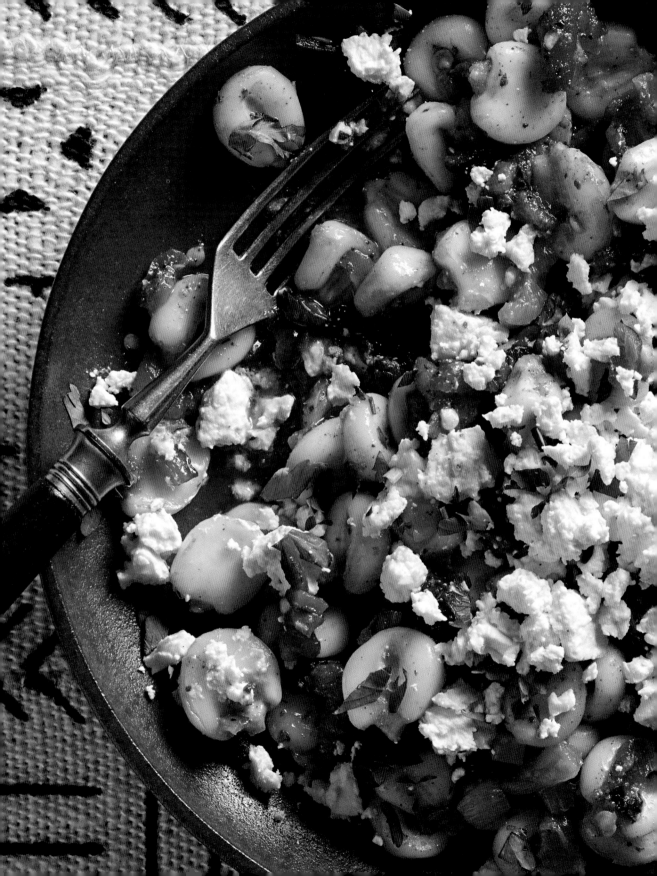

FOR THE PAPRIKA VINAIGRETTE

2 tablespoons avocado oil

Juice of 1 lemon (about 3 tablespoons)

2 garlic cloves, grated with a Microplane

1 teaspoon fine sea salt

1 teaspoon sweet paprika with oil

1 teaspoon dried oregano

1 teaspoon garlic powder

¼ teaspoon freshly ground black pepper

4. MAKE THE VINAIGRETTE: In a large bowl, whisk together the avocado oil, lemon juice, grated garlic, salt, sweet paprika, oregano, garlic powder, and pepper.

5. Once the peppers have cooled, peel off the charred exterior with your fingers. The moisture from the container should make it easier. Remove and discard the seeds and ribs from the bell peppers, poblano, and jalapeño, depending on how spicy you want it.

6. Stack the roasted peppers and cut into thin slices, then into 1-inch pieces. Add the peppers to the dressing and stir to evenly coat them.

7. Drain the hominy and add it to the large bowl while still warm. Toss everything together to fully combine.

8. Garnish with the feta, cilantro, and parsley. Store any leftovers in an airtight container in the fridge for 3 to 5 days.

green lentil salad

Every now and then, I challenge myself to make a green salad that is delicious, nutritious, and different than any other salad I've made before. With this one—if I say so myself—I really knocked it out of the park. I opened my fridge and looked at what I had, and just kept adding—but every ingredient is well worth it. This salad has everything you need for a filling, satisfying meal: hearty kale and lentils, crunchy cucumbers and snap peas, nutty pumpkin seeds, and olives that taste just like butter. But the real star of it all is the warm dressing made right in the pan that softens the vegetables and gives the dish an incredible garlicky flavor.

To save time, chop your vegetables and prepare the pumpkin seeds and lentils in advance (you can store the veggies in the fridge in a plastic bag with a damp paper towel). The base will keep for several days, but serving the dressing warm is an absolute must. **SERVES 8 TO 10**

1 cup uncooked green lentils

1 bunch lacinato kale, stems removed, leaves cut into small pieces (see page 251)

10 Brussels sprouts, shredded with a mandoline (about 1½ cups)

1 bunch scallions, trimmed, white and light green parts cut into ¼-inch slices

¼ cup Castelvetrano olives, sliced

2 Persian cucumbers (or half an English cucumber, seeded), chopped into confetti-size pieces

⅔ cup snap peas, trimmed and cut into ¼-inch pieces on a bias

½ cup pumpkin seeds

1. In a medium pot, bring 4 cups of water to a boil over high heat. Rinse and pick over the lentils and add to the pot. Cook until al dente, 20 to 30 minutes. Drain the lentils.

2. While the lentils cook, combine the kale, Brussels sprouts, scallions, olives, cucumbers, and snap peas in a large bowl.

3. In a large skillet over medium heat, toast the pumpkin seeds. Don't leave these unattended! Every so often, pick up the pan and shake the seeds around so they don't burn. Remove the pan from the heat when the seeds have turned brown and have a nutty, fragrant aroma, 5 to 7 minutes.

(continued)

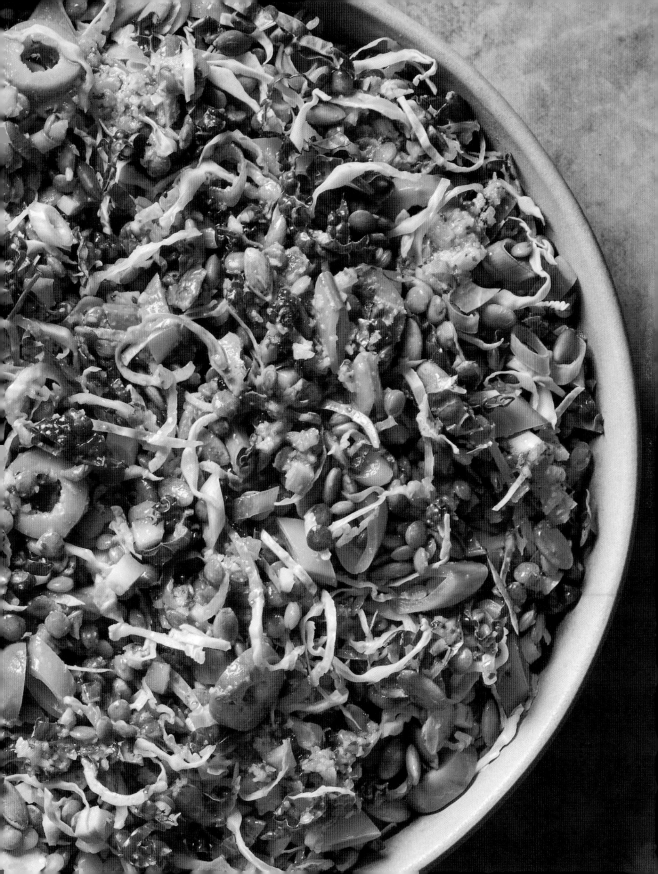

⅓ cup extra virgin olive oil

1 large (or 2 small) shallot, finely chopped

1 teaspoon fine sea salt, plus more to taste

6 medium garlic cloves, minced

1 teaspoon dried oregano

½ teaspoon garlic powder

½ teaspoon onion powder

3 lemons

2 tablespoons rice vinegar

¼ teaspoon freshly ground black pepper

2 tablespoons nutritional yeast (optional)

4. MAKE THE DRESSING: Heat the olive oil in a large skillet over medium-low heat. Add the shallot and sauté until translucent, 3 to 4 minutes.

5. Season with ½ teaspoon of the salt. Once the shallots are softened, add the minced garlic to the pan. Sauté for another 3 to 4 minutes, until fragrant—be careful not to burn it. Tip: Don't skip this step! If you don't cook the garlic enough, it has too much of a bite. I love a bit of brown for a deeper, more caramelized taste.

6. Take the pan off the heat and add the oregano, garlic powder, and onion powder.

7. Juice the lemons directly into the pan. Add the rice vinegar, the remaining ½ teaspoon salt, the pepper, and nutritional yeast, if using. Adjust the seasonings to taste.

8. Add the lentils and pumpkin seeds to the greens and stir well to combine. Pour the warm dressing over the salad directly from the pan and mix everything together.

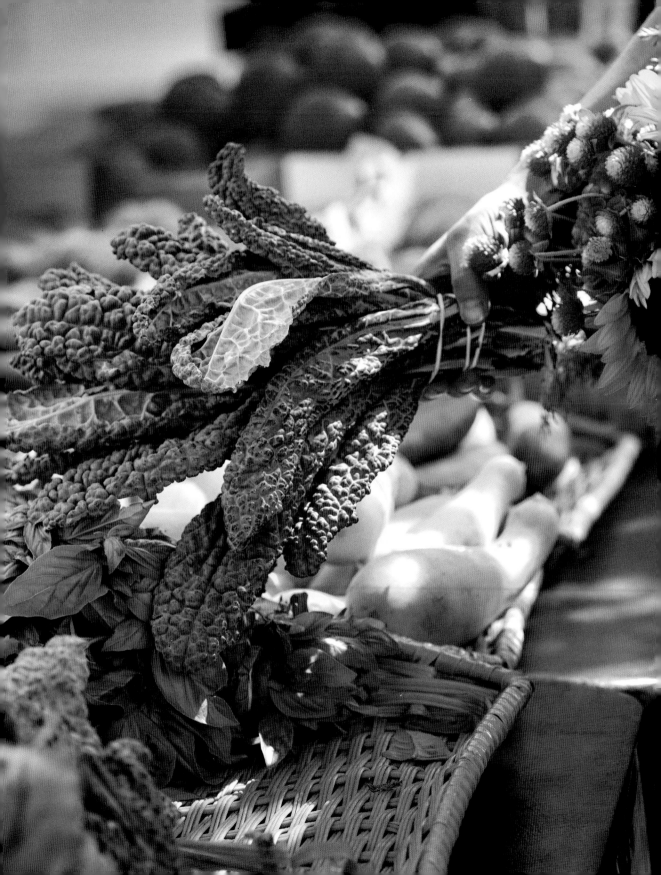

orzo pasta salad

By sautéing the onions, peppers, mushrooms, and zucchini in this dish, you tease out the flavors of the veggies to create a mouthwatering juice that brings everything together. Pouring the warm veggies over the spinach, olives, and artichokes slightly wilts the spinach and brings all ingredients to the perfect temperature. The next time you sign up to bring pasta salad to a party, you'll thank me! **SERVES 8**

1 teaspoon fine sea salt, plus more to taste

1 cup uncooked orzo

2 tablespoons plus 1 teaspoon extra virgin olive oil, plus more as needed

½ red onion, finely chopped

½ red bell pepper, finely chopped

2 garlic cloves, chopped

½ cup baby bella mushrooms, stemmed and cut into quarters

5 baby zucchini, or 2 medium zucchini, cut into ¼-inch-thick coins

Half of a (6.5-ounce) jar artichoke hearts marinated in oil, drained and cut into bite-size pieces

¼ cup Kalamata olives, chopped

½ cup fresh baby spinach

½ cup ciliegine (small mozzarella balls)

FOR THE DRESSING

⅓ cup extra virgin olive oil

Juice of 2 lemons (about ⅓ cup)

¼ cup red wine vinegar

¼ cup white miso paste

⅓ cup nutritional yeast

1 tablespoon dried oregano

2 garlic cloves, grated with a Microplane

½ teaspoon fine sea salt

1. Boil a large pot of water and season with the salt. Cook the orzo according to package directions and drain.

2. While the pasta cooks, heat 1 tablespoon of the olive oil in a medium pan over medium heat. Sauté the onion until translucent, about 5 minutes, then add the bell pepper. Cook until the onion has browned slightly and the peppers are soft, another 5 to 7 minutes. Season with a pinch of salt. Add these vegetables to a large bowl.

3. Add another tablespoon of olive oil to the pan as needed and add the garlic and mushrooms. Cook until the mushrooms are slightly softened but still firm, about 5 minutes, and season with another pinch of salt. Add to the bowl with the peppers and onion.

4. Heat the remaining 1 teaspoon olive oil in the pan and sauté the zucchini for a few minutes on each side, until it has browned. Add to the bowl with the other vegetables. Stir in the artichoke hearts and olives. Add the pasta and baby spinach to the bowl and gently stir to combine.

5. MAKE THE DRESSING: Whisk together the olive oil, lemon juice, vinegar, miso, nutritional yeast, oregano, garlic, and salt in a small bowl until well combined.

6. Pour the dressing over the salad and mix well to make sure everything is evenly coated.

7. Fold in the mozzarella once the pasta has cooled to room temperature and season to taste. Store leftovers in the fridge in an airtight container for 3 to 5 days.

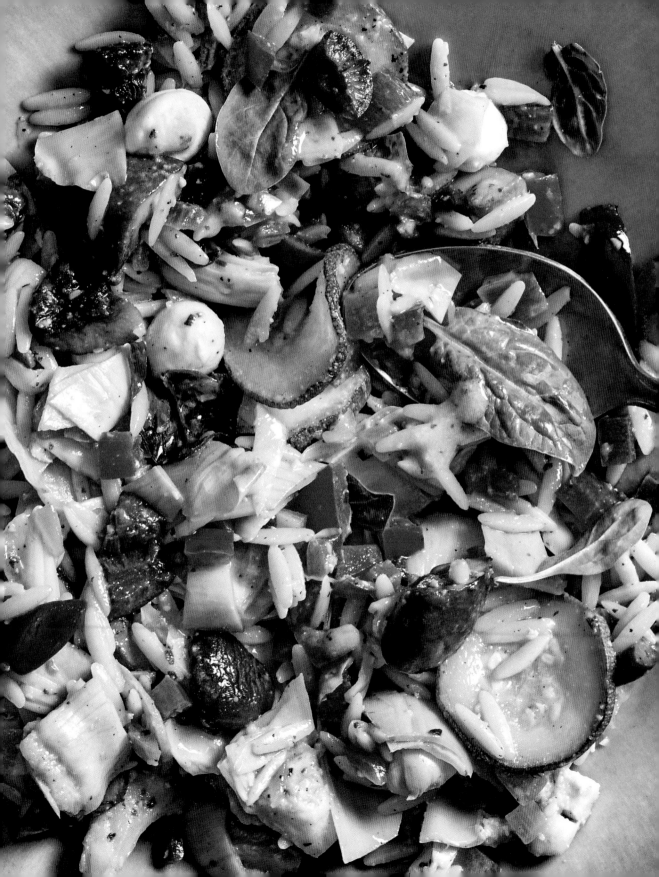

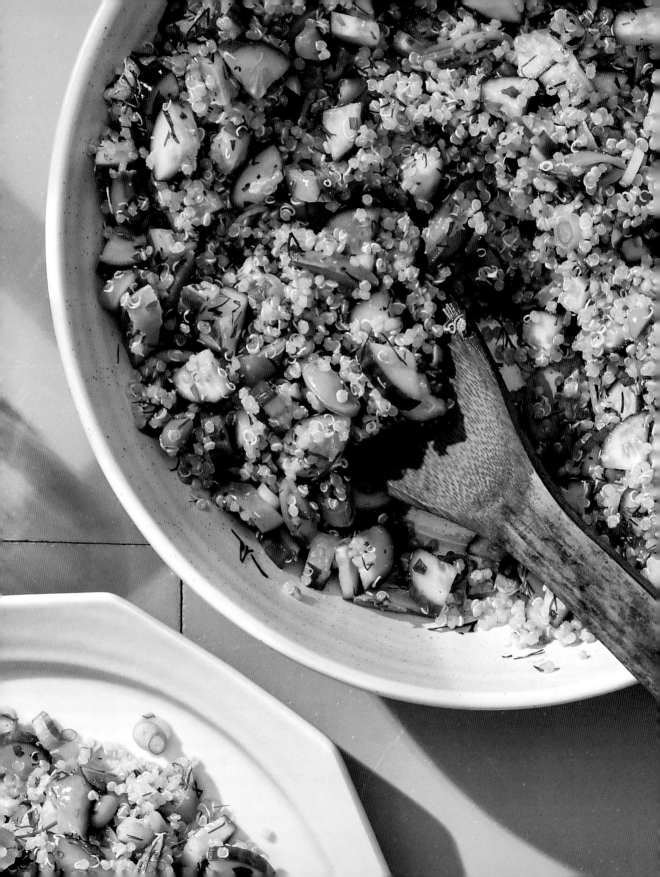

herby quinoa

I prefer eating quinoa as an ingredient in a dish rather than on its own. Balancing the filling grain with crunchy greens and an herby vinaigrette helps this salad check all the boxes. Plus, my best friend eats only gluten- and dairy-free foods, so quinoa gives me a natural way to create a delicious meal for her that everyone loves.

I dreamed this recipe up in the spring, when our nearby market was overflowing with snap peas, cucumbers, and bunches of scallions as long as my arm. Fortunately, all of the ingredients can also easily be found year-round. Protein-dense quinoa seemed like the perfect complement to those seasonal greens, since it kept the salad focused on my bounty but was still satisfying. The dressing makes it feel bright and herbaceous, a fitting taste to welcome delicious spring flavors. I love this salad in place of a pasta salad when entertaining, or if you just want to try out something new in the kitchen. **SERVES 4 TO 6**

1 cup uncooked quinoa

½ teaspoon fine sea salt, plus more to taste

2 cups snap peas, trimmed and cut into ¼-inch pieces on a bias

1 bunch scallions, trimmed, light green and white parts cut into ¼-inch slices

6 Persian cucumbers, chopped

FOR THE HERBY VINAIGRETTE

¼ cup extra virgin olive oil

Juice of 2 lemons (about ⅓ cup)

1 teaspoon garlic powder

1 tablespoon rice vinegar

1 teaspoon fine sea salt

¼ teaspoon freshly ground black pepper

¼ cup chopped fresh dill or cilantro

¼ cup chopped fresh parsley

1. Rinse the quinoa in a fine-mesh strainer under cold water and drain well. Place the quinoa in a large saucepan and cover with 2 cups water. Season with the salt and place over medium heat. Cook for 15 minutes, or until a small white tail (the germ) comes out of each grain. Cover the quinoa for 5 minutes, then uncover the saucepan and fluff with a fork. Let the quinoa come to room temperature (or cool for as long as you can).

2. Add the cooked quinoa to a large bowl and combine with the snap peas, scallions, and cucumbers.

3. MAKE THE VINAIGRETTE: Whisk together the olive oil, lemon juice, garlic powder, rice vinegar, salt, pepper, dill, and parsley in a small bowl until well combined.

4. Pour the dressing over the greens and quinoa and mix to evenly coat. Season to taste. Store any leftovers in the fridge in an airtight container for 3 to 5 days.

caramelized tomato & leeks with arugula

I love any excuse to cook up caramelized onions, and these flavorful, pan-seared leeks are the perfect way to enjoy a similar flavor profile in a salad. The combination of warm, roasted tomatoes and leeks is both comforting and impressive. It's a total showstopper, especially if you're looking for a well-rounded meal that can be served tableside, right in the pan. You can use any kind of tomatoes you have, but I recommend smaller ones—they have so much more flavor and you can find them in a variety of colors. **SERVES 4**

1 teaspoon fine sea salt

1 cup dried Israeli couscous

⅓ cup extra virgin olive oil

2 leeks, cleaned, trimmed, and cut into 1-inch discs

1 cup cherry tomatoes

2 lemons

1 teaspoon dried oregano

1 teaspoon garlic powder

¼ teaspoon freshly ground black pepper

2 cups arugula

¼ cup pine nuts

1 cup crumbled feta

Fresh parsley, to garnish

1. Add 4 cups of water to a large pot and season with ½ teaspoon of the salt. Place over high heat and bring to a boil. Add the couscous and cook for 7 to 8 minutes, until al dente. Drain and return to the pot while you prepare the rest of the salad.

2. Heat the olive oil in a large pan over medium heat. After 2 to 3 minutes, or once the oil shimmers, add the leeks. Cook the leeks until they start to brown, 2 minutes on each side, using tongs or a fork to turn them over. Once the leeks are seared, lower the heat to prevent them from burning.

3. Add the tomatoes to the pan. Cook the leeks and tomatoes, flipping occasionally, until they caramelize, 8 to 10 minutes. Remove the leeks and tomatoes from the pan.

4. Remove the pan from the heat. Juice the lemons directly into the pan and whisk together with the olive oil that remains in the pan. Add the oregano, garlic powder, remaining ½ teaspoon salt, and the pepper and whisk to combine.

5. Add the cooked couscous to the pan and stir so it's evenly coated in the dressing. Stir in the arugula.

6. Toast the pine nuts in a small pan over medium heat until fragrant and golden brown, stirring constantly so they don't burn, 5 to 7 minutes.

7. To serve, spoon the couscous and arugula mixture into a bowl and top with the leeks and tomatoes. Garnish with the feta, toasted pine nuts, and parsley.

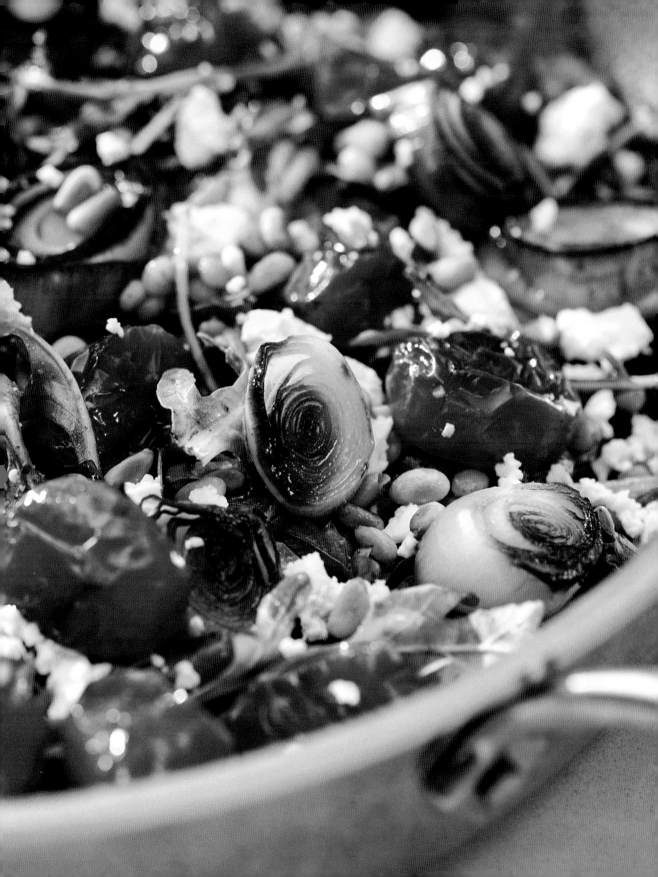

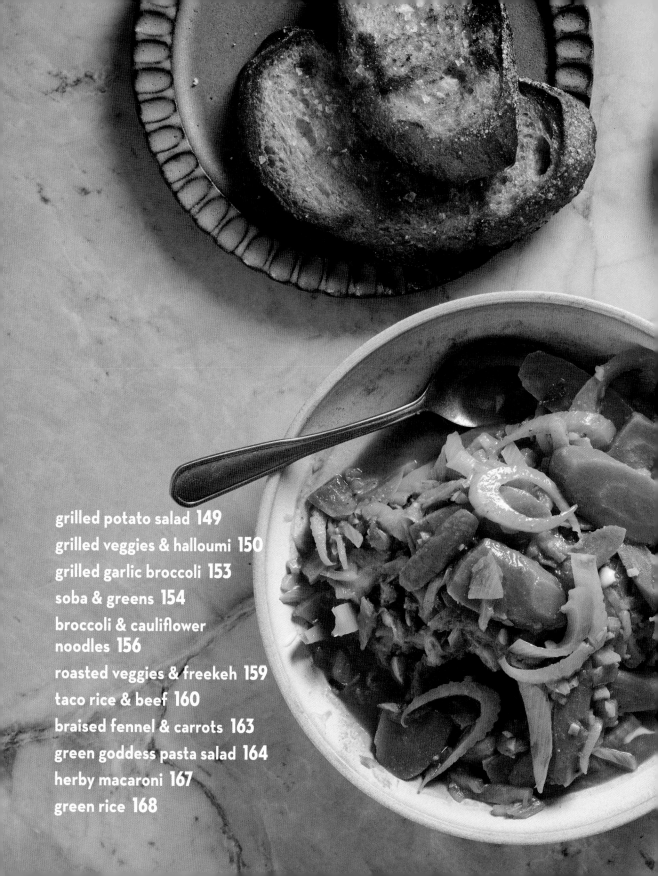

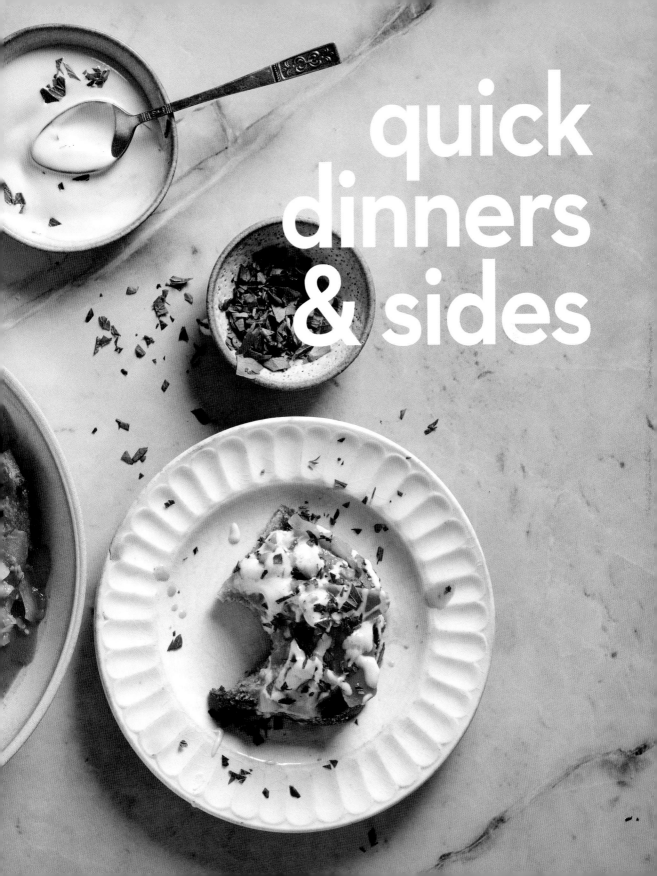

quick
dinners
& sides

I can't tell you how often I find myself rushing home from work, stressed about getting dinner on the table for my family. As someone who spends most of the day thinking about their next meal, I feel an added pressure to deliver something delicious for everyone. The recipes in this section are some of my go-tos when time is tight and I want a fulfilling meal for me and my family.

These aren't five-minute meals, but they're easy to prepare and often use few ingredients. It might take a little longer the first time you make these, but they're so simple to work into your regular dinner rotation when you're craving something delicious and nutritious. You can easily turn a side into a main by adding a bit of protein, or make a variety of your favorites when you invite friends for dinner. I hope these recipes inspire you the next time you're in a cooking rut or rushing home from work, craving nourishment.

" The recipes in this section are some of my go-tos when time is tight and I want a fulfilling meal for me and my family. "

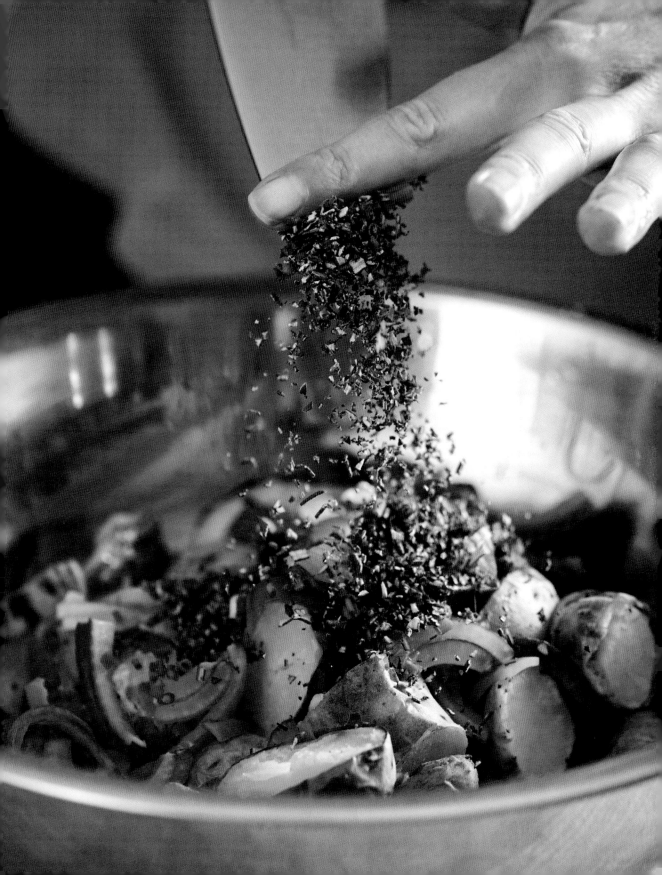

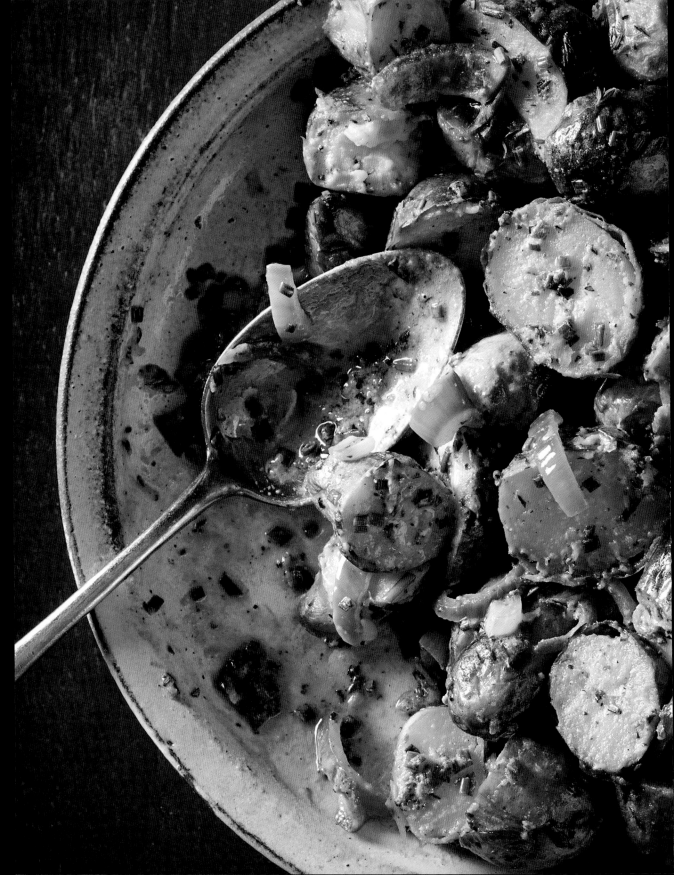

grilled potato salad

For a few years after we founded Baked by Melissa, my brother and I lived a block away from each other in Chelsea. He had a huge outdoor space at his apartment, so naturally I went there all the time for barbecues. He was a bachelor back then, so I became the de facto host of those gatherings—and as the host, I needed easy, fast recipes that didn't make a mess. This is that recipe. You can use any fresh herbs you have for the dressing—the greener you can make this, the better it will be. But make sure to use small baby potatoes so they get perfectly cooked inside and crispy outside. The grilled onions add a sweet, caramelized onion flavor, and I like to think the allium-filled aromas find the potatoes while they all cook together on the grill. This is best enjoyed standing over a grill while you wait for everything else to finish cooking. **SERVES 4 TO 6**

Two 24-ounce bags baby red potatoes

1 red onion, cut in half

FOR THE DRESSING

Juice of 2 lemons (about ⅓ cup)

⅓ cup extra virgin olive oil

2 tablespoons German mustard

¼ teaspoon freshly ground black pepper

1 teaspoon fine sea salt

2 tablespoons red wine vinegar

¼ cup nutritional yeast

1 tablespoon chopped fresh rosemary

1 teaspoon chopped fresh thyme

¼ cup finely chopped fresh chives

2 large garlic cloves, minced

1. Heat a grill pan or preheat a grill to medium-high heat.

2. Place the whole potatoes and red onion on the grill or grill pan. Cook for 20 minutes, turning occasionally with tongs so they cook evenly and don't burn, until the potatoes are cooked through and the onion has softened, then remove from the grill. While still hot, carefully cut the potatoes in half and carefully chop the red onion into ½-inch pieces.

3. MAKE THE DRESSING: Whisk together the lemon juice, olive oil, mustard, pepper, salt, vinegar, nutritional yeast, rosemary, thyme, chives, and garlic in a large bowl.

4. While the potatoes and onion are still warm, add them to the bowl with the dressing and gently stir until everything is evenly coated.

grilled veggies & halloumi

Whenever we grill meat for dinner, I always grill vegetables, too. I love how much a grill can transform the flavor of produce, so this dish needs only a drizzle of balsamic and lemon juice to wow your taste buds. You can use any vegetables you'd like, though I'd recommend sturdy vegetables like squash and peppers, so they don't fall through the grates. If you don't have a grill, a grill pan works just as well—as long as you're patient enough to get nicely charred grill marks.

SERVES 4 TO 6

1 medium zucchini

6 baby bella mushrooms

2 trumpet mushrooms

1 red bell pepper

One 8.8-ounce package halloumi

2 tablespoons avocado oil, plus more as needed

½ teaspoon fine sea salt

1 tablespoon balsamic vinegar

Juice of ½ lemon (about 1½ tablespoons)

1. Heat a grill pan or preheat a grill to medium-high heat.

2. Prep your veggies. Cut the zucchini into planks about ½ inch thick. Remove the stems from the baby bella mushrooms. Cut the ends off the trumpet mushrooms and cut in half lengthwise. Cut the cheeks off the red bell pepper.

3. Add all the veggies and halloumi to a large bowl and cover with the avocado oil. Add the salt and toss to evenly combine.

4. Carefully place the veggies and halloumi on the hot grill or grill pan. Cook for 5 minutes, or until grill marks begin to form. Flip with tongs and cook for about 5 more minutes. Depending on the size of your grill, you may need to cook in batches.

5. Once the veggies and halloumi are all cooked, cut them into smaller, bite-size pieces, collecting any cooking juices and adding them to a large bowl.

6. Add all the vegetables and halloumi to the bowl. Drizzle with the balsamic vinegar and lemon juice. Serve immediately.

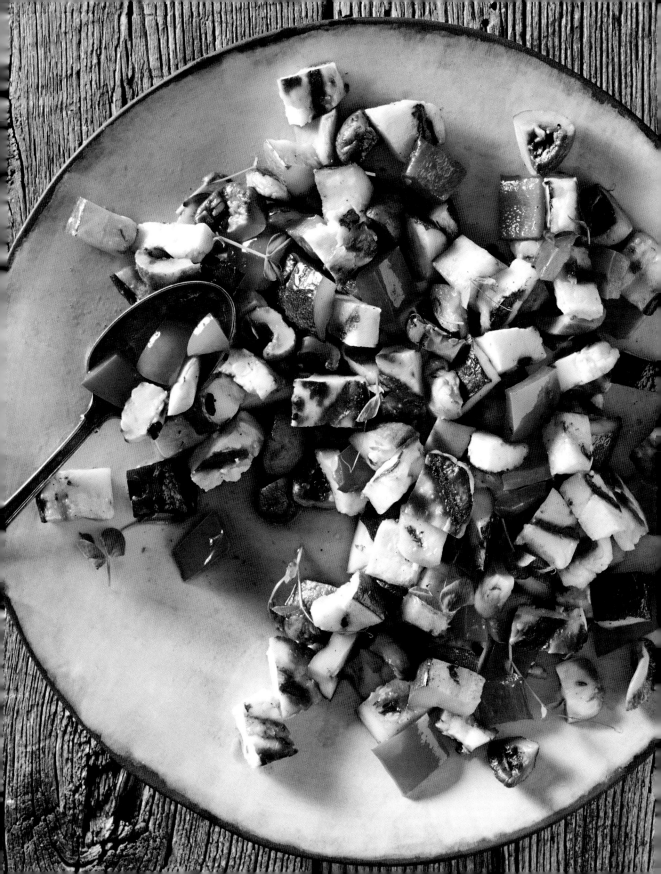

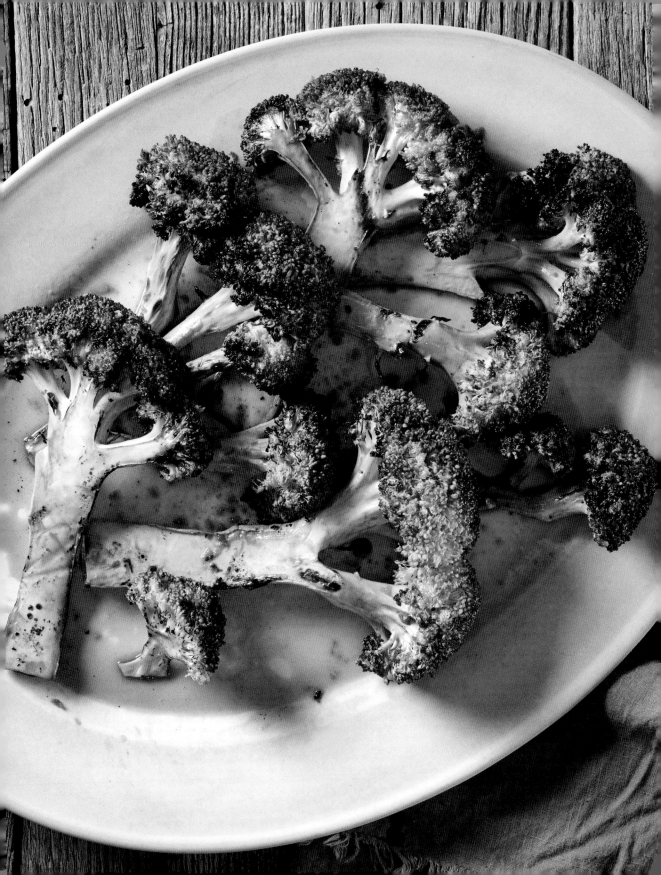

grilled garlic broccoli

At this point, it feels like I should start referring to Adi as my muse rather than my husband, since he has had so much influence over my cooking. Anyway, my muse went through a vegan phase a few years ago, which made me rethink how I made some of our favorite foods. Instead of grilled steaks, we tried steak-size slices of broccoli smothered in a tangy, savory marinade you'll want to eat like soup. It's no steak, but it made us forget about a ribeye in the moment. **SERVES 4 TO 6**

2 heads broccoli

FOR THE MARINADE

¼ cup regular soy sauce

2 tablespoons extra virgin olive oil

2 tablespoons toasted sesame oil

Juice of 1 lemon (about 3 tablespoons)

1 teaspoon honey

1 teaspoon minced ginger

3 garlic cloves, grated with a Microplane

1 tablespoon rice vinegar

¼ teaspoon freshly ground black pepper

1. Heat a grill pan or preheat a grill to medium-high heat.

2. Peel the stems of the broccoli (I use a Y peeler) to get off the hard exterior, the bottom of the stem, and any leaves. Cut the broccoli lengthwise, so you have palm-size slices.

3. MAKE THE MARINADE: Whisk together the soy sauce, olive oil, sesame oil, lemon juice, honey, ginger, garlic, rice vinegar, and pepper in a large bowl. Add the broccoli and gently stir to evenly coat the slices with the marinade.

4. Place the broccoli on the hot grill or grill pan and cook for 5 to 6 minutes. Flip and grill for another 5 to 6 minutes, until tender and grill marks appear. Transfer the broccoli back to the bowl to soak up more of the marinade. Serve warm.

soba & greens

The first time I made this salad, it was an accident. I had nothing in the fridge and was left riffling through the frozen veggies we had in the freezer, which at the time included broccoli, spinach, and edamame. I grabbed some soba noodles from the pantry because those are a guaranteed win for my kids. They add a bit more substance than other pastas, and with a quick peanut butter dressing, voilà—an easy, delicious recipe that's now on constant rotation in my house. **SERVES 2 TO 4**

1¼ teaspoons fine sea salt

Half of a 9.5-ounce package soba noodles

1 tablespoon avocado oil or other neutral oil

1 cup frozen broccoli

⅔ cup frozen shelled edamame

1 garlic clove, grated with a Microplane

1 head fresh spinach, chopped (around 3 cups)

1 bunch scallions, trimmed, light green and white parts cut into ¼-inch slices

Sesame seeds

FOR THE DRESSING

2 tablespoons toasted sesame oil

1 tablespoon rice vinegar

¼ cup creamy peanut butter

1 teaspoon grated ginger

Juice of 1 lemon (about 3 tablespoons)

3 tablespoons regular soy sauce

1. Fill a medium saucepan with water and add 1 teaspoon of the salt. Bring to a boil.

2. Add the soba noodles to the pot and cook for 4 to 5 minutes, until al dente. Drain the noodles and run them under cold water to prevent them from sticking together.

3. In a large sauté pan, heat the avocado oil over medium heat. Add the broccoli, edamame, and garlic to the pan. Add the remaining ¼ teaspoon salt and cook until the vegetables are thawed and slightly browned, 10 to 15 minutes.

4. MEANWHILE, MAKE THE DRESSING: Whisk together the sesame oil, rice vinegar, peanut butter, ginger, lemon juice, and soy sauce in a small bowl.

5. Combine the spinach and scallions in a medium bowl. Add the soba noodles and sautéed veggies to the bowl and stir together.

6. Pour the dressing on top and toss to combine. Garnish with sesame seeds. Store any leftovers in the fridge in an airtight container for 3 to 5 days.

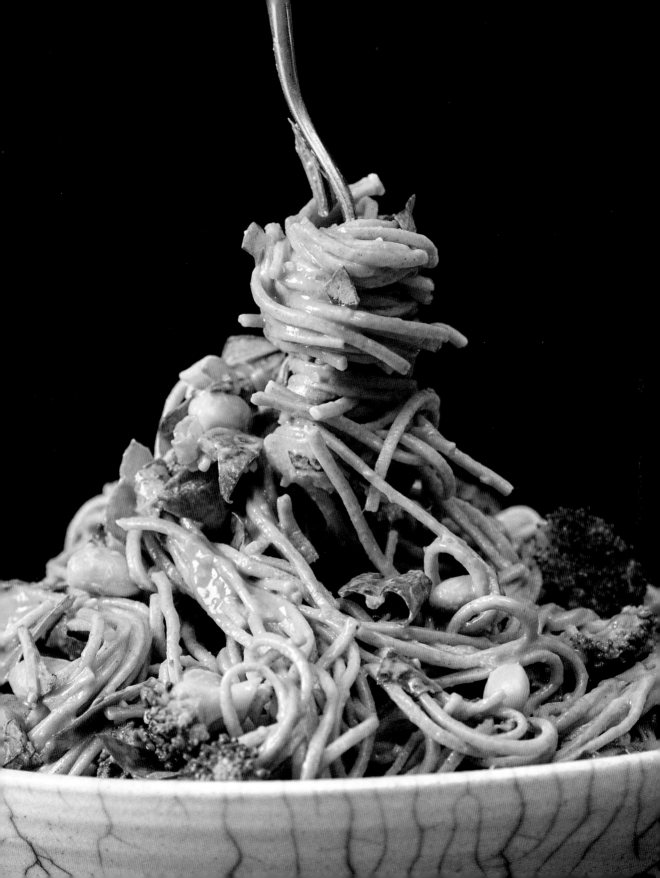

broccoli & cauliflower noodles

This recipe revitalizes our go-to veggies for an easy weeknight meal. The silky peanut dressing complements tender broccoli and cauliflower, the nuts and seeds give it extra crunch, and the best part is that dinner can be on the table in thirty minutes. **SERVES 4 TO 6**

One 8-ounce package pho rice noodles

1 head broccoli

⅓ to ½ of a large head cauliflower

½ cup snap peas, trimmed

1 bunch scallions, trimmed, light green and white parts cut on the bias into ¼-inch slices

¼ cup roasted salted cashews or peanuts, chopped

2 tablespoons sesame seeds

FOR THE DRESSING

¼ cup natural peanut butter, melted

2 garlic cloves, grated with a Microplane

2 tablespoons sesame oil

¼ cup plus 1 tablespoon regular soy sauce

Juice of 1½ lemons (about ¼ cup)

½ teaspoon garlic powder

1. Boil 3 cups of water in a kettle and place the rice noodles in a large bowl. Pour the hot water over the noodles and swirl with a wooden spoon. Let the noodles soak until tender, 6 to 9 minutes. Drain the noodles and rinse with cold water so they don't stick together.

2. Boil a large pot of water over high heat and prepare an ice bath.

3. Peel the broccoli stems with a Y peeler and trim the bottoms off. Peel the leaves off the cauliflower.

4. Add the broccoli, cauliflower, and snap peas to the pot and cook for 1 to 2 minutes, so they still have a crunch. Remove from the pot and transfer to the ice bath to stop the cooking. Let cool for several minutes.

5. Finely chop the broccoli and cauliflower and add them to a large bowl—you should have about 3 cups of each.

6. Cut the snap peas on the bias into ¼-inch pieces. Add the snap peas and scallions to the bowl.

7. Add the cashews and sesame seeds to a skillet over medium heat. Cook until fragrant and golden brown, tossing occasionally so they don't burn, 3 to 5 minutes.

8. MAKE THE DRESSING: In a medium bowl, whisk together the peanut butter, grated garlic, sesame oil, soy sauce, lemon juice, and garlic powder, whisking fully after adding each ingredient so the mixture stays smooth and the peanut butter doesn't harden.

9. Pour the dressing over the vegetables and stir to evenly coat. To serve, plate the rice noodles first, then top with the salad. Garnish with the toasted sesame seeds and cashews.

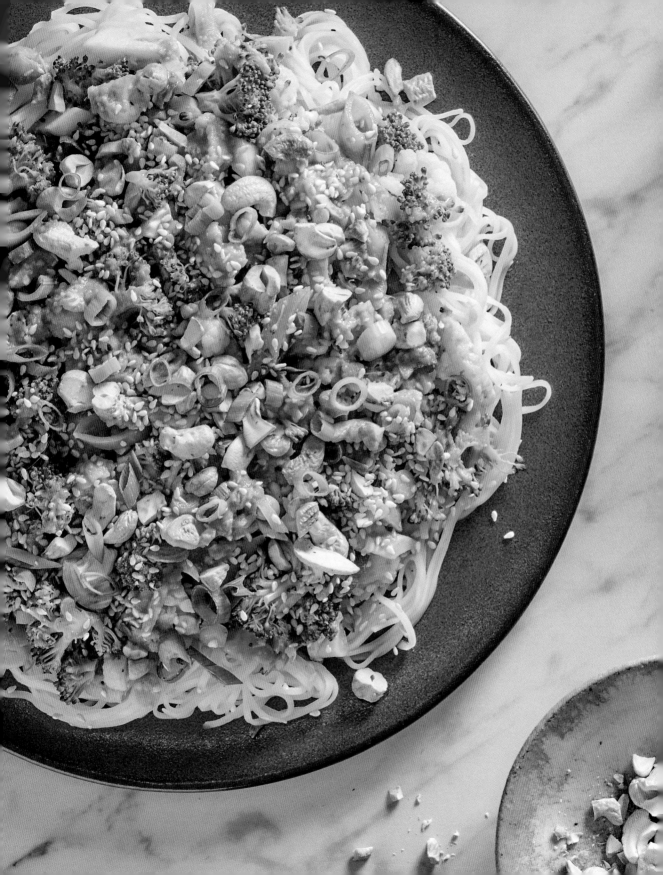

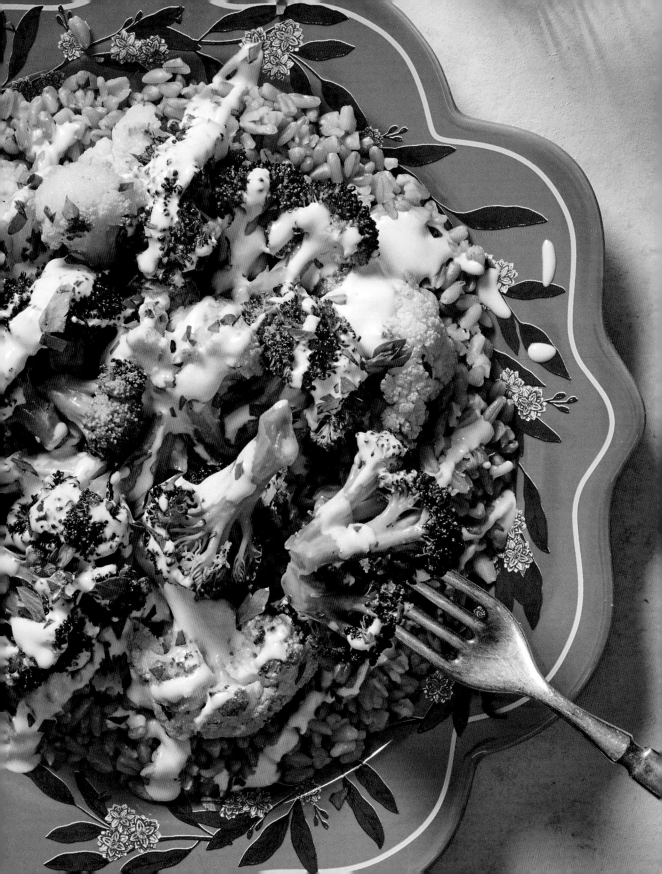

roasted veggies & freekeh

Adi and I used to make this for dinner at least once a week after busy days at work. It's so simple, nutritious, and delicious—all components of the perfect meal. By adding the herbs and garlic when the veggies have already cooked, the flavors are so much more powerful and don't become muted by the heat of the oven. I love the nuttiness and added nutrients that freekeh provides—the small ancient grain is commonly used in Middle Eastern cuisine and is packed with protein and fiber. To round out the meal, give it a quick, generous drizzle of tahina. **SERVES 4**

1 cup uncooked cracked freekeh

1 head cauliflower, chopped into 2-inch florets

¼ cup avocado oil

1 teaspoon fine sea salt

½ teaspoon freshly ground black pepper

1 head broccoli, chopped into 2-inch florets

FOR THE DRESSING

3 tablespoons extra virgin olive oil

Juice of 1 lemon (about 3 tablespoons)

2 tablespoons finely chopped fresh parsley

2 tablespoons finely chopped fresh cilantro

1 garlic clove, grated with a Microplane

Fine sea salt and freshly ground black pepper

Tahina

1. Cook the freekeh according to package instructions.

2. Preheat the oven to 420°F and line a baking sheet with parchment paper.

3. Toss the cauliflower with 2 tablespoons of the avocado oil in a large bowl until fully coated. Season with ½ teaspoon of the salt and ¼ teaspoon of the pepper.

4. Lay the cauliflower in a single layer on the baking sheet and roast for 15 minutes.

5. Meanwhile, toss together the broccoli florets with the remaining 2 tablespoons avocado oil in a large bowl. Season with the remaining ½ teaspoon salt and ¼ teaspoon pepper.

6. Remove the cauliflower from the oven and add the broccoli to the pan. Roast the broccoli and cauliflower together for 30 more minutes, until tender and lightly golden brown.

7. MAKE THE DRESSING: Whisk together the olive oil, lemon juice, parsley, cilantro, and garlic. Season with salt and pepper to taste.

8. Once the broccoli and cauliflower are ready, toss them in the dressing to evenly coat. Serve the roasted cauliflower and broccoli over the freekeh and drizzle with tahina.

taco rice & beef

My family loves tacos (I mean, who doesn't?). Taco rice and beef are easy, approachable ingredients I know my kids will eat and love, and together, they're pretty much a guaranteed home run. The rice cooks with the beef almost like a risotto, soaking up all the spices and seasonings to make it extra flavorful. I like to make these a little greener than traditional tacos by serving them in little gem lettuce cups. You can also save any leftovers for quesadillas, burritos, or a burrito bowl. Top these tacos with your favorite ingredients—I like avocado, sour cream, and fresh herbs—for an easy weeknight meal. Just don't add salt until the end, because taco seasonings have different spice and salt levels depending on the brand. **SERVES 6**

2 tablespoons extra virgin olive oil

1 small yellow onion, chopped

4 garlic cloves, chopped

1 pound ground beef (I recommend 85/15 fat content)

⅓ cup uncooked long-grain rice

2 tablespoons tomato paste

1½ cups vegetable broth

2 tablespoons taco seasoning (I like Garden of Eatin')

Fine sea salt, to taste

Fresh parsley and cilantro, to garnish

Little gem lettuce, to serve

Ripe avocado, to serve

Sour cream, to serve

Lime wedges, to serve

1. Heat the olive oil in a large pan over medium heat. Add the onion and cook until translucent, 5 to 7 minutes. Stir occasionally so it doesn't burn.

2. Add the garlic to the pan and stir until fragrant, about 1 minute.

3. Add the beef to the pan and break up with a wooden spoon. After about 8 to 10 minutes, once the meat is mostly cooked (it's okay to still see some pink), stir in the rice and cook for 1 to 2 minutes.

4. Add the tomato paste and cook for 1 to 2 minutes to caramelize. Pour in the vegetable broth and lower the heat to a simmer. Cover and cook, stirring occasionally, until the liquid has been mostly absorbed, 15 to 20 minutes.

5. Add the taco seasoning and stir. Season to taste and garnish with parsley and cilantro. Serve in lettuce cups with avocado and sour cream, and a squeeze of lime if desired.

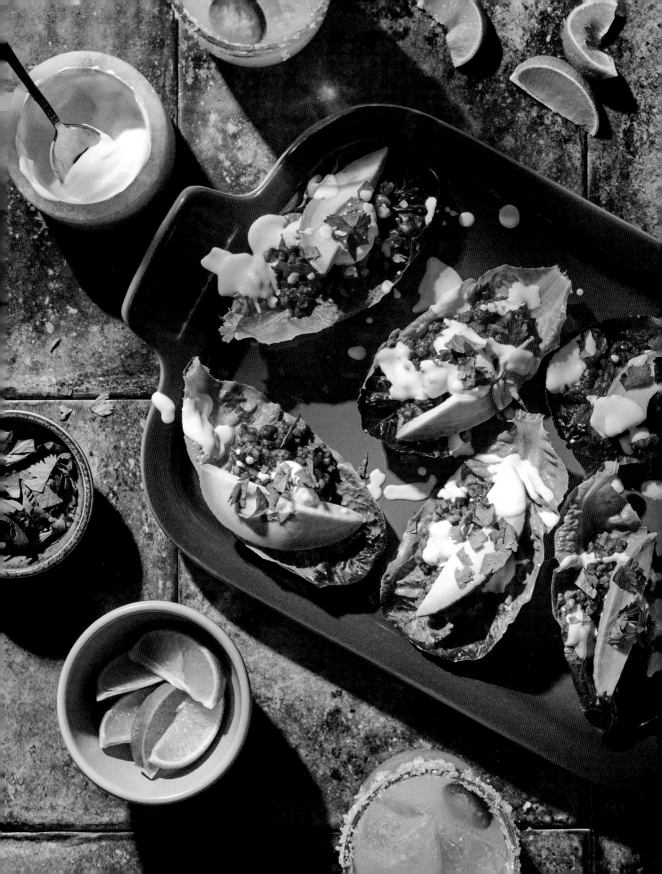

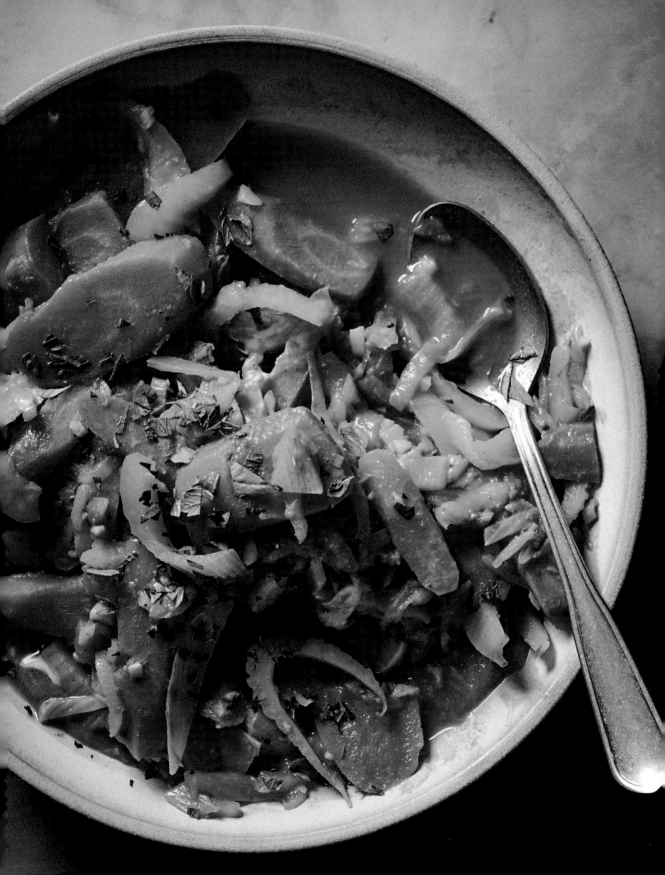

braised fennel & carrots

As he did with the Raw Fennel Salad (page 33), Adi made this warming, comforting dish for me every week when I was breastfeeding. This is also a magical dish when you aren't feeling well, like chicken soup for people who love vegetables. The ingredients have powerful healing benefits: turmeric, fennel, and carrots all reduce inflammation and contain heart-healthy antioxidants. Make the most of it and enjoy with bread toasted in extra virgin olive oil and topped with tahina, or serve as a side dish to your favorite protein. **SERVES 2 TO 4**

3 tablespoons extra virgin olive oil

1 medium yellow onion, sliced

2 bulbs fennel, trimmed and sliced, avoiding the core

4 medium carrots, peeled and cut on the bias into ½-inch pieces

4 to 6 garlic cloves, chopped

1½ teaspoons turmeric

1 teaspoon ground cumin

1 teaspoon fine sea salt

½ teaspoon freshly ground black pepper

2 cups vegetable broth

Juice of ½ lemon (about 1½ tablespoons)

1 tablespoon chopped fresh parsley

1. Heat the olive oil in a large skillet over medium heat. Add the onion, fennel, and carrots to the pan and cook, stirring occasionally, until the onions are translucent, 10 to 12 minutes.

2. Stir in the garlic and continue to cook until fragrant, 1 to 2 minutes.

3. Add the spices and seasonings to the pan and toast them for about 1 minute. Pour in the vegetable broth, cover, and let simmer for 15 minutes, or until the carrots are fork-tender. Lower the heat if the liquid starts to boil.

4. Remove the lid and cook to reduce the broth as desired (for less broth, cook uncovered for a little longer), 5 to 7 minutes.

5. Add the lemon juice right before removing the pan from the heat. Garnish with the parsley and serve. Store any leftovers in the fridge in an airtight container for 3 to 5 days.

green goddess pasta salad

You know how much I love the color green. This pasta salad combines the one I grew up eating with my Green Goddess Salad (page 98), and let me tell you, whenever I make it for friends and family, it's the first dish to go. If you're not immediately captivated by the bright green while you make this, you will be when you take your first bite. The broccolini adds texture, the bits of olives lend a salty bite, and the thick, creamy dressing is almost entirely basil and spinach, giving the salad a burst of nutrients and a pop of color. **SERVES 6**

FOR THE DRESSING
Juice of 2 lemons (about ⅓ cup)
¼ cup extra virgin olive oil
2 tablespoons rice vinegar
1 cup fresh basil leaves
1 cup fresh spinach
2 garlic cloves
1 small shallot, peeled
¼ cup raw, unsalted cashews
⅓ cup nutritional yeast
1 teaspoon fine sea salt
Handful of fresh chives (optional)

One 13.2-ounce package fusilli pasta, cooked according to package directions, drained, and cooled to room temperature
1 cup pitted Castelvetrano olives, chopped
1 cup snap peas, trimmed and chopped
1 bunch scallions, trimmed, light green and white parts cut into ¼-inch slices
2 bunches broccolini, blanched and chopped into 1-inch pieces (3 to 4 cups)
7 ounces ciliegine (small mozzarella balls), cut in half, a few reserved for garnish
Fresh basil leaves, to garnish

1. MAKE THE DRESSING: Add the lemon juice, olive oil, and rice vinegar to a large high-powered blender and pulse to combine. Add the basil, spinach, garlic, shallot, nuts, nutritional yeast, salt, and chives, if using, and pulse again, until smooth.

2. Toss together the cooked pasta, olives, snap peas, scallions, broccolini, and mozzarella in a large bowl.

3. Pour the dressing over the pasta and stir until everything is evenly coated.

4. Garnish with fresh mozzarella and fresh basil. Store any leftovers in the fridge in an airtight container for 3 to 5 days.

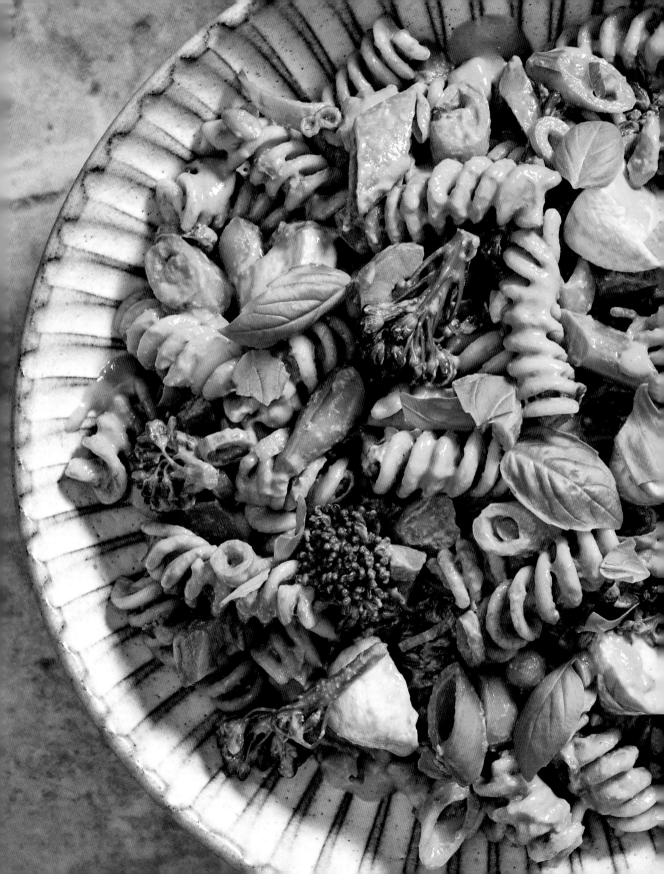

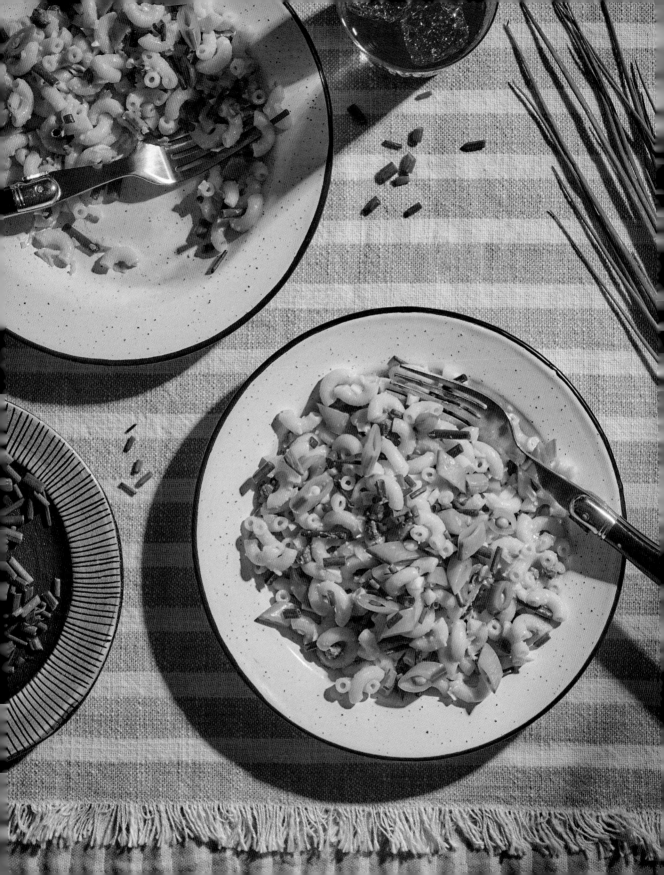

herby macaroni

Growing up, the only macaroni salad I knew was the kind that came in those little containers from the deli. I can't say I loved that macaroni salad, but whenever it was included in the order, I had to at least take a bite of it. Something I do love, though, is to re-create classic dishes from my childhood. My take is greener, fresher, and filled with nutrients, all held together with a creamy vegan Caesar dressing. You can mix and match whatever greens you have on hand and make it your own for a delicious, nostalgic meal. **SERVES 6**

FOR THE VEGAN CAESAR DRESSING

¼ cup extra virgin olive oil

1 tablespoon Dijon mustard

Juice of 2 to 3 lemons (about ⅓ to ½ cup)

⅓ cup plain hummus

2 tablespoons whole capers, plus 2 tablespoons brine

¼ cup capers, chopped

3 garlic cloves, grated with a Microplane

1 teaspoon fine sea salt

⅓ cup nutritional yeast

1 tablespoon rice vinegar

1 pound elbow macaroni, cooked according to package instructions, and still warm

1 cup chopped green cabbage, cut into confetti-size pieces

1 cup snap peas, cut into ½-inch pieces on a bias

⅓ cup finely chopped fresh chives, plus more for garnish

1. MAKE THE DRESSING: Whisk together the olive oil, mustard, lemon juice, hummus, whole capers and brine, chopped capers, garlic, salt, nutritional yeast, and rice vinegar in a small bowl.

2. Stir three-quarters of the dressing into the hot pasta—this will help soften the garlic flavor.

3. Add the cabbage, snap peas, and chives and stir to combine.

4. Pour in the remaining dressing and stir. Garnish with chives. Store any leftovers in the fridge in an airtight container for 3 to 5 days.

green rice

green rice I love the simplicity of plain white rice. In my quest to add nutrient-dense ingredients to some of my all-time favorite dishes without repeating the same thing over and over again, I landed on this bright, refreshing—and even crunchy—GREEN rice.

As in other green rice recipes you can find around the world, lemon juice and fresh herbs add so much to this dish. The key to getting the perfect bite with this recipe is cutting the broccoli to be the same size as the rice, so that each forkful is balanced with greens and rice. This could be considered a starchy side, so after I toss it all together with a simple vinaigrette, I like to serve it alongside proteins and more greens. **SERVES 6**

1 cup uncooked long-grain white rice

1 large head broccoli

1 bunch fresh cilantro, finely chopped

1 bunch fresh flat-leaf parsley, finely chopped

FOR THE DRESSING

Juice of 2 lemons (about ⅓ cup)

¼ cup extra virgin olive oil

1 large or 2 small garlic cloves, grated with a Microplane

1 tablespoon rice vinegar

1 teaspoon fine sea salt

1. Cook the rice according to package instructions.

2. Bring a large pot of water to boil. Prepare an ice bath and have nearby. Peel the stems of the broccoli with a Y peeler and trim off the ends. Blanch the broccoli in the boiling water for about 3 minutes, then immediately transfer to the ice bath to stop the cooking.

3. Once the broccoli is cool, finely chop it so each piece is about the size of a grain of rice.

4. MAKE THE DRESSING: Whisk together the lemon juice, olive oil, garlic, rice vinegar, and salt in a small bowl.

5. In a large bowl, combine the rice, broccoli, and herbs. Pour in the vinaigrette and stir until everything is evenly mixed. Store any leftovers in the fridge in an airtight container for 3 to 5 days.

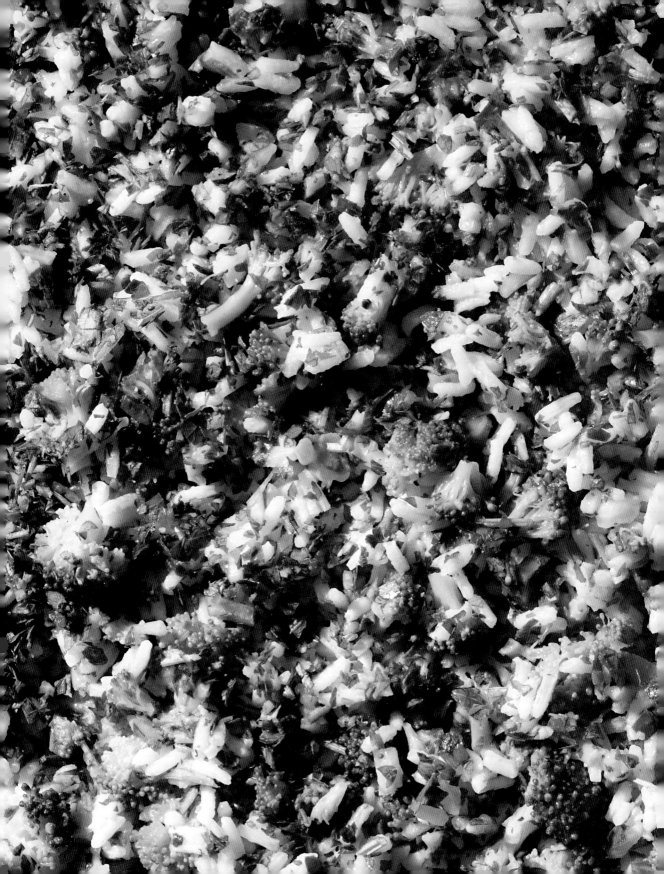

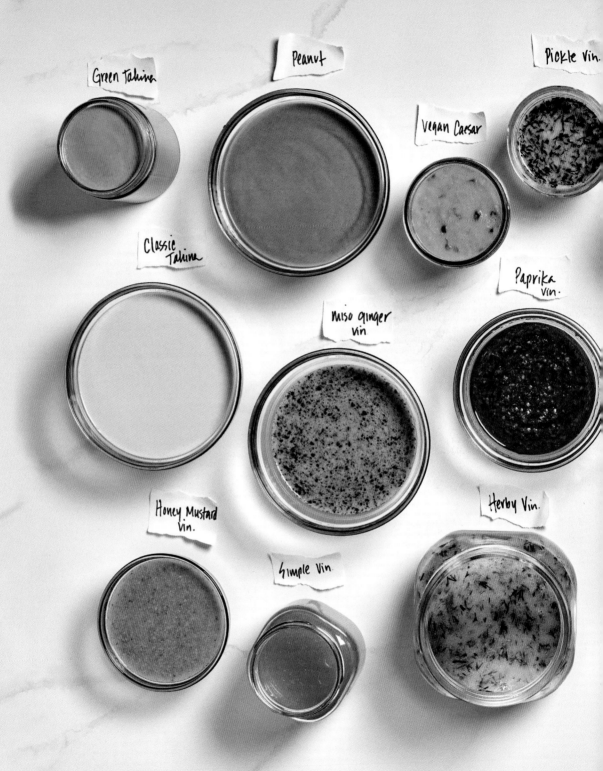

Green Tahini

Peanut

Pickle Vin.

Vegan Caesar

Classic Tahina

Paprika Vin.

Miso ginger vin.

Honey Mustard Vin.

Herby Vin.

Simple Vin.

Garlic Vin.

Tahina Vin.

Vegan Pesto

Miso Vin.

Herby Tahina

Vegan Ranch

Italian Vin.

Creamy Honey mustard

Green Goddess

dressings

vinaigrettes

simple vinaigrette

MAKES ⅔ CUP

Juice of 2 lemons (about ⅓ cup)
¼ cup extra virgin olive oil
1 large or 2 small garlic cloves, minced
1 tablespoon rice vinegar
1 teaspoon fine sea salt
¼ teaspoon freshly ground black pepper

1. Whisk together the lemon juice, olive oil, garlic, rice vinegar, salt, and pepper in a small bowl or jar until emulsified.

2. Store in the fridge in a sealed jar for up to 1 week.

miso vinaigrette

MAKES 1½ CUPS

⅓ cup extra virgin olive oil
Juice of 2 lemons (about ⅓ cup)
¼ cup red wine vinegar
¼ cup white miso paste
⅓ cup nutritional yeast
1 tablespoon dried oregano
2 garlic cloves, grated with a Microplane
½ teaspoon fine sea salt

1. Whisk together the olive oil, lemon juice, vinegar, miso paste, nutritional yeast, oregano, garlic, and salt in a small bowl or jar until emulsified.

2. Store in the fridge in a sealed jar for up to 1 week.

herby vinaigrette

MAKES 1 CUP

¼ cup extra virgin olive oil
Juice of 2 lemons (about ⅓ cup)
1 teaspoon garlic powder
1 tablespoon rice vinegar
1 teaspoon fine sea salt
¼ teaspoon freshly ground black pepper
2 tablespoons chopped fresh dill or cilantro
2 tablespoons chopped fresh parsley

1. Whisk together the olive oil, lemon juice, garlic powder, rice vinegar, salt, pepper, dill, and parsley in a small bowl or jar until emulsified.

2. Store in the fridge in a sealed jar for up to 1 week.

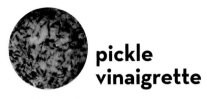

pickle vinaigrette

MAKES ¾ CUP

2 tablespoons chopped fresh dill

Juice of 2 lemons (about ⅓ cup)

⅓ cup extra virgin olive oil

1 tablespoon rice vinegar

2 garlic cloves, grated with a Microplane

½ teaspoon fine sea salt

1. Whisk together the dill, lemon juice, olive oil, rice vinegar, garlic, and salt in a small bowl or jar until emulsified.

2. Store in the fridge in a sealed jar for up to 1 week.

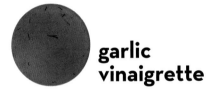

garlic vinaigrette

MAKES ½ CUP

Juice of 2 lemons (about ⅓ cup)

3 tablespoons extra virgin olive oil

1½ tablespoons (or a healthy splash) white vinegar

2 large garlic cloves, minced

¾ teaspoon fine sea salt

1. Whisk together the lemon juice, olive oil, vinegar, garlic, and salt in a small bowl or jar until emulsified.

2. Store in the fridge in a sealed jar for up to 1 week.

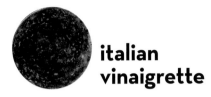

italian vinaigrette

MAKES 1 CUP

¼ cup red wine vinegar

⅓ cup extra virgin olive oil

Juice of 2 lemons (about ⅓ cup)

1 heaping teaspoon dried oregano

½ teaspoon garlic powder

½ teaspoon onion powder

1 heaping teaspoon chopped fresh parsley

2 large garlic cloves, grated with a Microplane

1 teaspoon fine sea salt

2 tablespoons nutritional yeast

¼ teaspoon freshly ground black pepper

1. Whisk together the vinegar, olive oil, lemon juice, oregano, garlic powder, onion powder, parsley, grated garlic, salt, nutritional yeast, and pepper in a small bowl or jar until emulsified.

2. Store in the fridge in a sealed jar for up to 1 week.

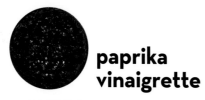

paprika vinaigrette

MAKES ⅓ CUP

2 tablespoons avocado oil

Juice of 1 lemon (about 3 tablespoons)

2 garlic cloves, grated with a Microplane

1 teaspoon fine sea salt

1 teaspoon sweet paprika with oil

1 teaspoon dried oregano

1 teaspoon garlic powder

¼ teaspoon freshly ground black pepper

1. Whisk together the avocado oil, lemon juice, grated garlic, salt, sweet paprika, oregano, garlic powder, and pepper in a small bowl or jar until emulsified.

2. Store in the fridge in a sealed jar for up to 1 week.

honey mustard vinaigrette

MAKES ¾ CUP

¼ cup extra virgin olive oil

2 tablespoons German mustard

2 teaspoons honey

Juice of 2 lemons (about ⅓ cup)

1 teaspoon fine sea salt

½ teaspoon freshly ground black pepper

1. Whisk together the olive oil, mustard, honey, lemon juice, salt, and pepper in a small bowl or jar until emulsified.

2. Store in the fridge in a sealed jar for up to 1 week.

creamy dressings

vegan pesto

MAKES 1 CUP

2 cups fresh basil leaves

Juice of 1½ lemons (about ¼ cup)

3 tablespoons extra virgin olive oil

1 teaspoon fine sea salt

2 garlic cloves

⅓ cup pine nuts

½ cup nutritional yeast

1. Add the basil, lemon juice, olive oil, salt, garlic, pine nuts, and nutritional yeast to a food processor or blender and blend until combined.

2. Store in the fridge in a sealed jar for 3 to 5 days.

creamy miso-ginger vinaigrette

MAKES 1 CUP

3 garlic cloves

One 1-inch knob fresh ginger, peeled (about 2 teaspoons grated ginger)

¼ cup toasted sesame oil

¼ cup avocado oil or other neutral oil

2 tablespoons white miso paste

2 tablespoons rice vinegar

Juice of 2 lemons (about ⅓ cup)

¼ cup nutritional yeast

1 teaspoon fine sea salt

1. Add the garlic, ginger, sesame oil, avocado oil, miso, rice vinegar, lemon juice, nutritional yeast, and salt to a blender and process until smooth.

2. Store in the fridge in a sealed jar for up to 1 week.

green goddess

MAKES 1½ CUPS

1 cup fresh basil leaves

1 cup fresh spinach

2 garlic cloves

1 small shallot

Juice of 2 lemons (about ⅓ cup)

¼ cup extra virgin olive oil

¼ cup nuts of your choice (I used raw, unsalted cashews and walnuts)

⅓ cup nutritional yeast

1 teaspoon fine sea salt

2 tablespoons rice vinegar

Handful of fresh chives (optional)

1. Add the basil, spinach, garlic, shallot, lemon juice, olive oil, nuts, nutritional yeast, salt, rice vinegar, and chives, if using, to a blender and process until smooth.

2. Store in the fridge in a sealed jar for up to 1 week.

vegan caesar

MAKES 1 CUP

¼ cup plain hummus

1 teaspoon Dijon mustard

Juice of 2 lemons (about ⅓ cup)

2 garlic cloves, grated with a Microplane

2 tablespoons capers packed in brine, chopped, plus 1 tablespoon brine

1 teaspoon fine sea salt

3 tablespoons extra virgin olive oil

⅓ cup nutritional yeast

1. Whisk together the hummus, mustard, lemon juice, garlic, capers, caper brine, salt, olive oil, and nutritional yeast in a small bowl until emulsified.

2. Store in the fridge in a sealed jar for up to 1 week.

vegan ranch

MAKES 1½ CUPS

Heaping ½ cup raw, unsalted cashews, plus more as needed

⅓ cup extra virgin olive oil

½ cup nutritional yeast

Juice of 2 lemons (about ⅓ cup)

1 tablespoon finely chopped fresh chives

1 tablespoon finely chopped fresh dill

1½ teaspoons garlic powder

1 teaspoon onion powder

¾ teaspoon fine sea salt

1. Add the cashews, olive oil, ¾ cup water, and nutritional yeast to a blender and pulse to combine. If needed, add more cashews until it reaches a creamy yogurt-like consistency.

2. Once smooth, pour into a large mason jar and add the lemon juice, chives, dill, garlic powder, onion powder, and salt. Stir together.

3. Store in the fridge in a sealed jar for up to 1 week.

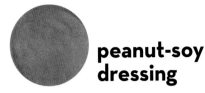

peanut-soy dressing

MAKES 1 CUP

¼ cup natural peanut butter, melted

2 garlic cloves, grated with a Microplane

2 tablespoons sesame oil

¼ cup plus 1 tablespoon regular soy sauce

Juice of 1½ lemons (just over ¼ cup)

½ teaspoon garlic powder

1. Whisk together the peanut butter, grated garlic, sesame oil, soy sauce, lemon juice, and garlic powder until smooth.

2. Store in the fridge in a sealed jar for up to 1 week.

creamy honey mustard

MAKES 1 CUP

⅓ cup mayonnaise

⅓ cup Dijon mustard

2 tablespoons honey

1 teaspoon fine sea salt

Juice of ½ lemon (about 1½ tablespoons)

1. Whisk together the mayo, mustard, honey, salt, and lemon juice in a small bowl until smooth.

2. Store in the fridge in a sealed jar for 3 to 5 days.

tahina-based dressings

green tahina

MAKES 2 CUPS

1 bunch fresh parsley

1 bunch fresh cilantro

4 garlic cloves

Juice of 2 lemons (about ⅓ cup)

1 teaspoon fine sea salt

1 cup tahina

1. Add the parsley, cilantro, garlic, lemon juice, ½ cup cold water, and the salt to a blender and pulse until the liquid turns green.

2. Pour in the tahina and blend until smooth.

3. Add water as needed until you reach a consistency that can be drizzled.

4. Store in the fridge in a sealed jar for up to 1 week.

classic tahina

MAKES 1½ CUPS

½ cup tahina

Juice of 3 lemons (a bit more than ½ cup)

3 garlic cloves, grated with a Microplane

1 teaspoon fine sea salt

1. Stir together the tahina and ½ cup cold water until the mixture is smooth and pourable but not too runny. It'll look like it's separating at first, but keep stirring! Add more water as needed, 1 teaspoon at a time, until it reaches a mustard-like consistency.

2. Add the lemon juice, garlic, and salt and stir to combine.

3. Taste and adjust the seasonings as desired.

4. Store in the fridge in a sealed jar for up to 1 week.

tahina vinaigrette

MAKES 1 CUP

½ cup tahina

2 tablespoons Dijon mustard

2 garlic cloves, grated with a Microplane

1 teaspoon fine sea salt

¼ teaspoon freshly ground black pepper

Juice of 2 lemons (about ⅓ cup)

1 tablespoon rice vinegar

2 teaspoons honey

1. Mix the tahina with ⅓ cup cold water. It's going to get thick, then it will get thinner. Add more water until the mixture reaches a mustard-like consistency.

2. Add the mustard, garlic, salt, pepper, lemon juice, rice vinegar, and honey. Whisk to combine.

3. Store in the fridge in a sealed jar for up to 1 week.

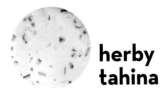

herby tahina

MAKES 2½ CUPS

1 cup tahina

Juice of 3 lemons (a bit more than ½ cup)

1½ tablespoons chopped fresh dill

¼ cup chopped fresh chives

2 garlic cloves, grated with a Microplane

1 teaspoon fine sea salt

1. In a large bowl, stir together the tahina and ¾ cup cold water until it reaches the desired consistency. It'll look like it's separating, but keep stirring! The ideal consistency is smooth and pourable but not too runny.

2. Add the lemon juice, dill, chives, garlic, and salt and stir to combine.

3. Store in the fridge in a sealed jar for up to 1 week.

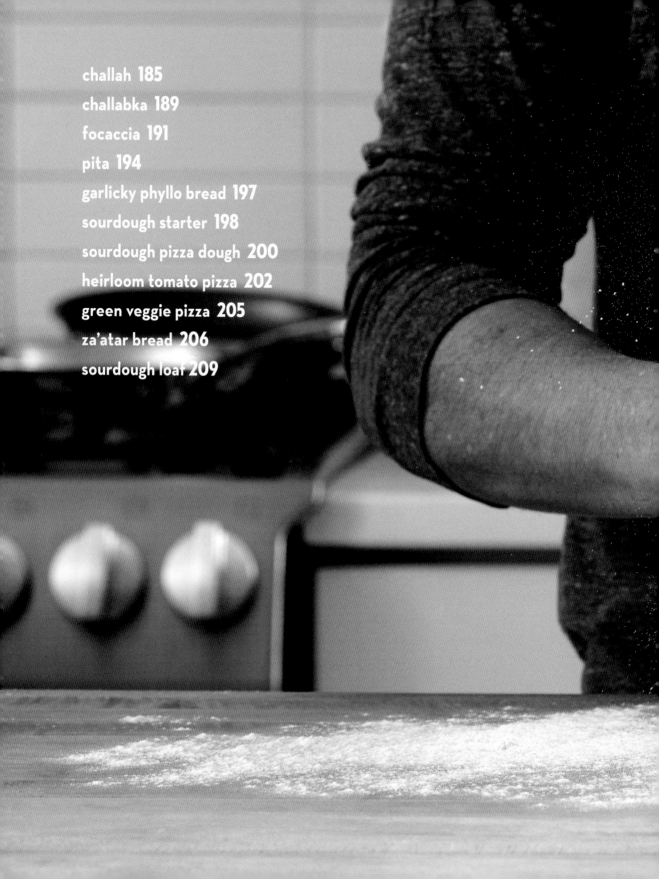

breads

If I walk into my house and Bob Marley is playing, I know Adi is cooking. In the kitchen, we're the dynamic duo. You can't eat just salads or vegetables—you need a healthy variety of all the most delicious foods to live a happy life. Adi is incredibly patient in the kitchen, so bread baking was meant for him. Everything he makes the girls call "Daddy's Famous" (Daddy's Famous Grilled Cheese, Daddy's Famous Egg Crêpes), but the breads he makes are truly incredible, so it's my privilege to share some of his favorite recipes here. There's no better way to enjoy a meal than with fresh bread on the side.

Growing up, Adi was a fairly picky eater. He admittedly ate a lot of chocolate—so much that now he hardly touches it!—and a lot of fresh, fluffy pita. While he didn't leap for the salads and small plates the way we do now, he spent years watching his parents and grandparents cook, absorbing the traditions of their Eastern European and North African heritages, shopping for colorful Mediterranean produce, and inhaling spiced, herbaceous aromas. Now, spending time cooking for his family is one of his greatest passions, which shouldn't come as a surprise—the kitchen is where we fell in love.

I should preface these recipes by saying we don't bake fresh bread all the time. But if you're looking for a showstopping Shabbat centerpiece or a fun activity on a cold winter day, fresh bread is the way to go.

A note about bread making: You'll notice that these recipes use metric measurements rather than imperial. Bread making is incredibly precise, so converting the following recipes into imperial measurements won't produce the same results. A good scale can be found inexpensively online (we got ours on Amazon) and is one of the best investments to make in a well-used kitchen.

" If you're looking for a showstopping centerpiece or a fun activity on a cold winter day, fresh bread is the way to go. "

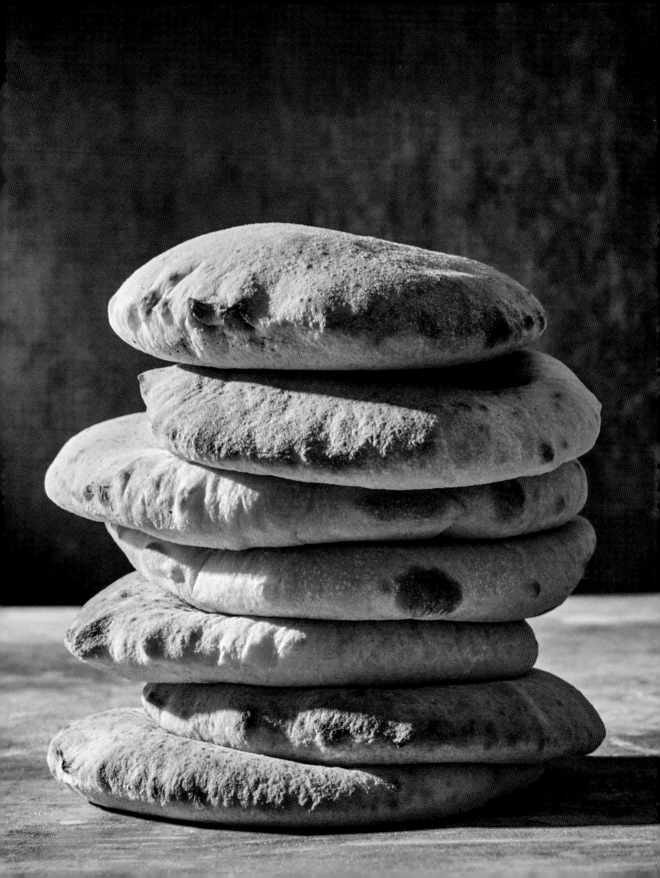

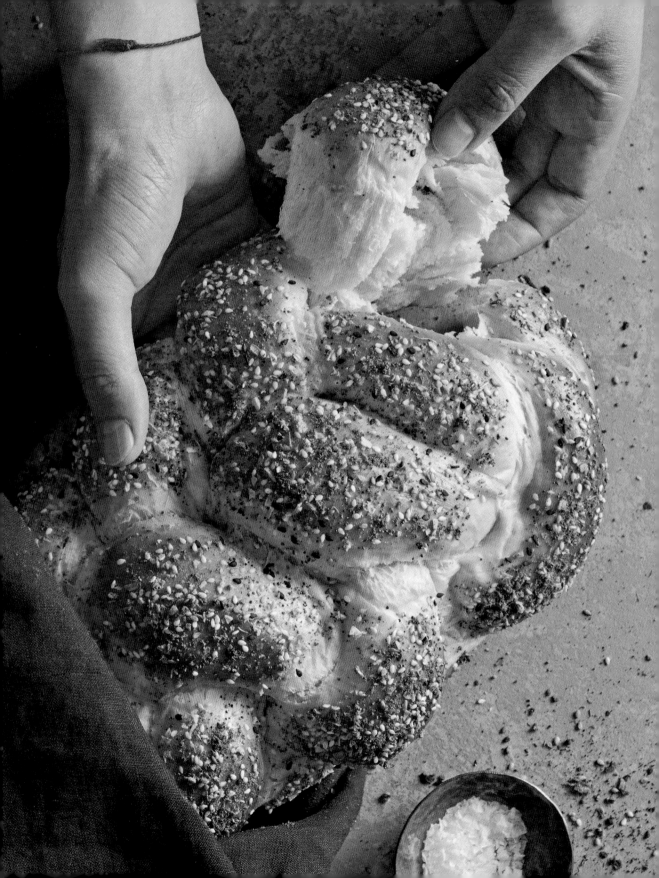

challah

Every Friday night, we have Shabbat dinner as a family. Adi and I both grew up Jewish and are raising our kids to be Jewish. But my childhood experience in New Jersey was so different from Adi's in Israel. There, the religion is the culture and there's a huge community of people sharing similar traditions. Adi has a deep respect and appreciation for those traditions, which I'm so lucky my girls get to experience.

You can't have a Shabbat without freshly made challah. The slightly sweet, soft bread makes a stunning centerpiece whether you make it sweet or savory and is a great way to get your kids involved in the kitchen. Plus, there are few things more fun than braiding strands of the pillowy dough. **MAKES 2 LOAVES**

FOR THE LEAVEN

9 grams instant yeast

10 grams sugar

FOR THE DOUGH

3 large eggs

20 grams honey

60 grams sugar

900 grams all-purpose flour, plus more for dusting

90 grams extra virgin olive oil, plus more for oiling the bowl

15 grams kosher salt

FOR TOPPING

1 large egg

2 tablespoons everything bagel seasoning

2 tablespoons za'atar

TO SERVE

Honey butter

Extra virgin olive oil

Flaky sea salt

1. MAKE THE LEAVEN: In a small bowl, whisk together the yeast, sugar, and 350 grams lukewarm (110°F to 115°F) water. Let sit for 5 to 10 minutes, until the top begins to bubble.

2. MAKE THE DOUGH: In the bowl of a stand mixer fitted with the whisk attachment, beat the eggs on medium speed until very fluffy. Turn the mixer to low and slowly add the yeast mixture. Once combined, add the honey and sugar.

3. Turn the mixer off and sift about one-third of the flour into the mixture. Mix on low until just combined. Switch out the whisk for the dough hook. Sift another one-third of the flour in and mix until just combined. Turn the mixer off again and sift in the remaining flour. Mix on low until the dough forms a smooth ball.

4. Add the olive oil and mix until just combined. Let rest for 10 to 15 minutes.

5. Repeat with the salt, and rest for 10 to 15 minutes more.

(continued)

6. Lightly oil a large bowl. Turn the dough out on a lightly floured surface and knead lightly to form a ball. Gently place the dough in the oiled bowl and turn so all the dough has a light coating of oil. Cover with plastic wrap and let rise until doubled in size, around 3 hours.

7. Line two baking sheets with parchment paper. Turn the dough out on a lightly floured surface and divide into twelve equal balls.

8. Roll each ball into a long strand, about 15 inches long.

9. Working on a large, flat surface, pinch six of the dough strands together at the top. Cross the strand farthest to the right over the other five strands.

10. Take the strand second from the left across the other four strands. Pull the outer left strand into the middle, so it's third from the left.

11. Cross the strand second from the right to the left side.

12. Pull the farthest right strand to the middle, so it's third from the right.

13. Repeat this process until you run out of dough and the challah is fully braided.

14. Repeat steps 9 through 13 with the remaining six strands of dough and carefully transfer the braided loaves to the baking sheets.

15. Cover the braided challah with plastic wrap and store in a warm place to let the loaves rise until doubled in size, about 45 minutes. While the dough rises, preheat the oven to 375°F.

16. TOP THE DOUGH: Beat the egg in a small bowl with 1 tablespoon water and use a pastry brush to brush it over the dough. Sprinkle the everything bagel seasoning and za'atar over the tops.

17. Bake the challah for 24 minutes, until golden brown with an internal temperature of 190°F, rotating the baking sheets after 12 minutes.

18. Remove the challah from the oven and transfer to a wire rack to cool. Serve with honey butter or salt and oil. Store the bread in a large ziplock bag to keep it fresh, and eat within 3 days.

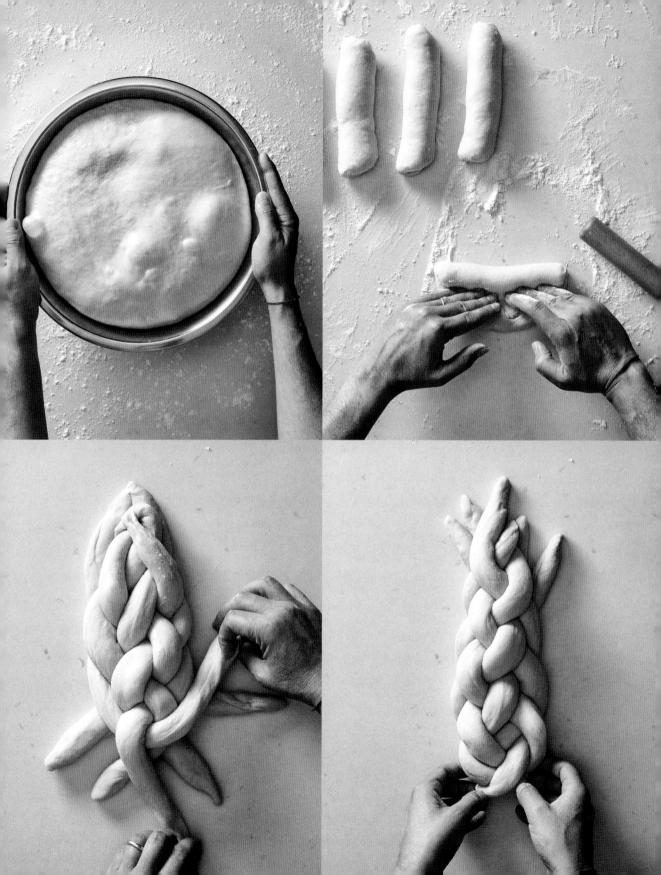

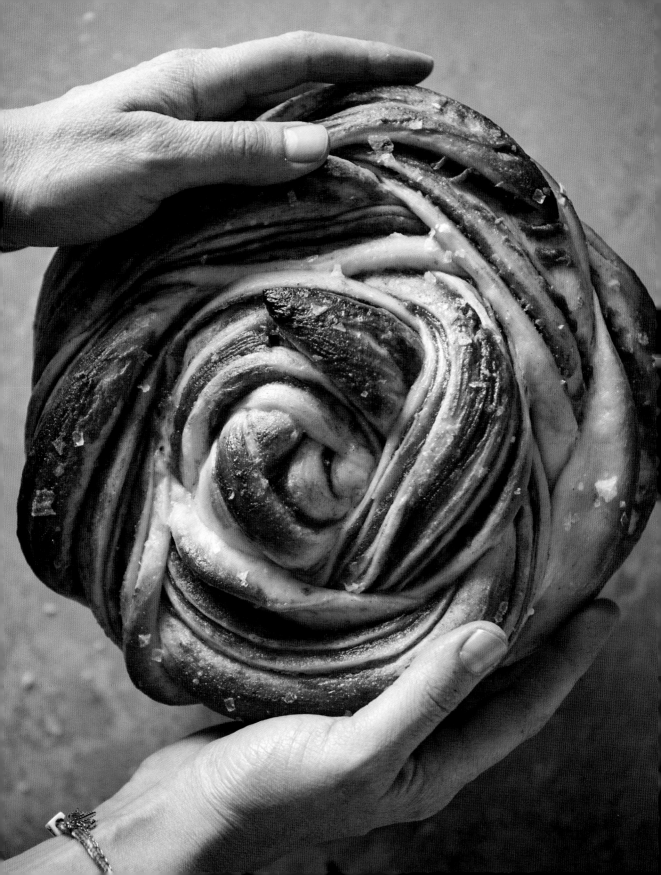

challabka

The challabka is a creation of my own making—it's a combination of soft challah and flavorful braided babka. Don't get me wrong, I love plain, fluffy challah. But for celebrations where you want to add to the festivities (like Rosh Hashanah, for example), a challah filled with twists and swirls of date caramel is absolutely the way to go. Like its braided cousin, the challabka can be time-consuming, but it's easy to make once you get the hang of it and will impress guests, no question. Don't limit yourself to date caramel as a filling, either—you could just as easily follow the same technique with spiced apples, chocolate, or cheese. **MAKES 2 LOAVES**

FOR THE LEAVEN
9 grams instant yeast
10 grams sugar

FOR THE DOUGH
3 large eggs
20 grams honey
60 grams sugar
900 grams all-purpose flour, plus more for dusting
90 grams extra virgin olive oil, plus more for oiling the bowl and rolling the dough
15 grams kosher salt

FOR THE FILLING AND TOPPING
2 cups Date Caramel (page 230)
1 teaspoon cinnamon
1 large egg
Sesame seeds

1. MAKE THE LEAVEN: In a small bowl, whisk together the yeast, sugar, and 350 grams lukewarm (110°F to 115°F) water. Let sit for 5 to 10 minutes, until the top begins to bubble.

2. MAKE THE DOUGH: In the bowl of a stand mixer fitted with the whisk attachment, beat the eggs on medium speed until very fluffy. Turn the mixer to low and slowly add the yeast mixture. Once combined, add the honey and sugar.

3. Sift about one-third of the flour into the mixture and mix on low. It will look like a creamy cake batter at this point. Switch to the dough hook, sift in another one-third of the flour, and mix until just combined. Turn off the mixer again and sift in the remaining flour. Mix on low until the dough forms a smooth ball.

4. Add the olive oil and mix until just combined. Let rest for 10 to 15 minutes.

5. Repeat with the salt, and rest for 10 to 15 minutes more.

6. Lightly oil a large bowl. Turn the dough out on a lightly floured surface and knead lightly to form a ball. Gently place the dough in the oiled bowl and turn so all the dough has a light coating of oil. Cover with plastic wrap and let rise until doubled in size, around 3 hours.

(continued)

7. Line two baking sheets with parchment paper. Turn the dough out on a lightly floured surface and divide into sixteen equal balls.

8. Roll each ball into a long strand, about 15 inches long.

9. MAKE THE FILLING: In a small bowl, stir together the date caramel and cinnamon.

10. On a lightly oiled surface, flatten one of the strands with a rolling pin. Spread 1 tablespoon of date caramel over the dough and roll it up lengthwise. Set aside and repeat with the remaining balls.

11. Start braiding. To make a round challabka, place two pairs of dough strands parallel to each other on a flat surface.

12. Take another pair and weave it under one dough strand and over the other, then repeat with another pair to create a hash sign.

13. Take the tails of the hash sign and work your way around the dough, tucking every other dough strand under the one to the left. Repeat this process until a wreath forms and you can tuck the ends of the dough underneath.

14. Repeat steps 11 through 13 with the remaining eight strands to create a second loaf.

15. Once the challabka are braided, place the loaves on the baking sheets and cover with plastic wrap to proof. Store in a warm place to let them rise until doubled in size, about 45 minutes. While the dough rises, preheat the oven to 375°F.

16. TOP THE DOUGH: Beat the egg in a small bowl with 1 tablespoon water and use a pastry brush to brush it over the dough. Sprinkle sesame seeds over the top.

17. Bake the challabka for 30 minutes, turning the baking sheets halfway through, until golden brown with an internal temperature of 190°F.

18. Remove the challabka from the oven and let cool on a wire rack before slicing. Store the bread in a large ziplock bag to keep it fresh, and eat within 3 days.

focaccia

Living in Hoboken means we're surrounded by the best Italian delis. The small New Jersey town is on the western edge of the Hudson River, with incredible views of the New York City skyline and cobblestone streets, and like most of New Jersey, it booms with Italian American culture. Fresh focaccia covered in veggies, garlic, and herbs is never hard to find, but if we always bought it, we'd miss out on the fun of making it (and eating it fresh from the oven).

So many breads are labor-intensive and precise, but focaccia makes me feel like a kid again. The dough is similar to pizza dough, but since it's left to rise, it develops big, fluffy bubbles inside. Making it is the best activity to do with kids—everyone can take turns pushing their fingers in the dough to create little nooks for the extra virgin olive oil to curl into. It's like Play-Doh. Add whatever veggies you have on hand and just sink into the process. It's a blast. **MAKES 1 FOCACCIA**

FOR THE LEAVEN

50 grams organic bread flour

50 grams T85 flour

100 grams active sourdough starter

FOR THE DOUGH

300 grams einkorn flour

450 grams organic bread flour

250 grams T70 flour

165 grams leaven

25 grams fine sea salt

Extra virgin olive oil

FOR TOPPING

Flaky sea salt

Cherry tomatoes

Scallions

Olives

Onions

Garlic cloves

Fresh herbs

Make the leaven the night before making the dough. For a 100 percent hydrated active starter fed at 4 p.m., make the leaven around 10 p.m.

1. MAKE THE LEAVEN: In a small bowl, mix together the bread flour, T85 flour, sourdough starter, and 100 grams room-temperature water. Cover and let rest overnight.

2. MAKE THE DOUGH: The following morning, combine the einkorn flour, bread flour, T70 flour, and 750 grams room-temperature water in a large bowl. Mix lightly by hand and let the dough rest, covered, for 30 to 60 minutes so the flour can hydrate.

3. Add the leaven and salt to the dough and mix vigorously with your hands. Once everything is incorporated, begin to stretch and fold the dough by pulling each edge up in quarters and folding from 2 o'clock to 7 o'clock. Repeat this process across the whole bowl.

(continued)

4. Scrape down the sides of the bowl, cover, and let rest for 15 minutes.

5. Uncover the dough and stretch and fold it again for 1 minute. Cover and let rest for another 15 minutes.

6. Repeat the process once more and let rest.

7. After 15 minutes, fold the dough over itself and transfer to a clean bowl.

8. Let rest, covered with a lid or plastic wrap, for at least 6 hours in a warm place, until the dough is doubled in size, smooth, and shiny with air bubbles on top.

9. Grease a baking sheet with about 2 tablespoons olive oil, making sure to cover the whole sheet.

10. Transfer the dough to the baking sheet. Cover with a towel and let rest for 40 minutes.

11. Preheat the oven to 500°F. Remove the towel and cover the dough with another 2 tablespoons olive oil. Using your fingers, indent the dough so the top is covered with holes. Sprinkle with flaky sea salt.

12. TOP THE DOUGH: Decorate with any vegetables of your choice. I like to use olives, tomatoes, artichokes, scallions, onions, garlic, and herbs.

13. Lower the temperature to 475°F and bake for 25 to 30 minutes, until the top is golden brown. Transfer the finished product to a wire rack to cool. Store in a large ziplock bag for up to 3 days.

note: This recipe calls for four different types of flour: bread flour, T85, T70, and einkorn. All can be found easily online and even in some organic grocery stores.

BREAD FLOUR: A high-protein flour, which gives loaves a chewy crumb and golden crust.

T85: A high-protein malted wheat flour favored for its older milling practices.

T70: A high-extraction bread flour preferred by artisan bread bakers.

EINKORN: An ancient grain with lower gluten content and a sweet taste.

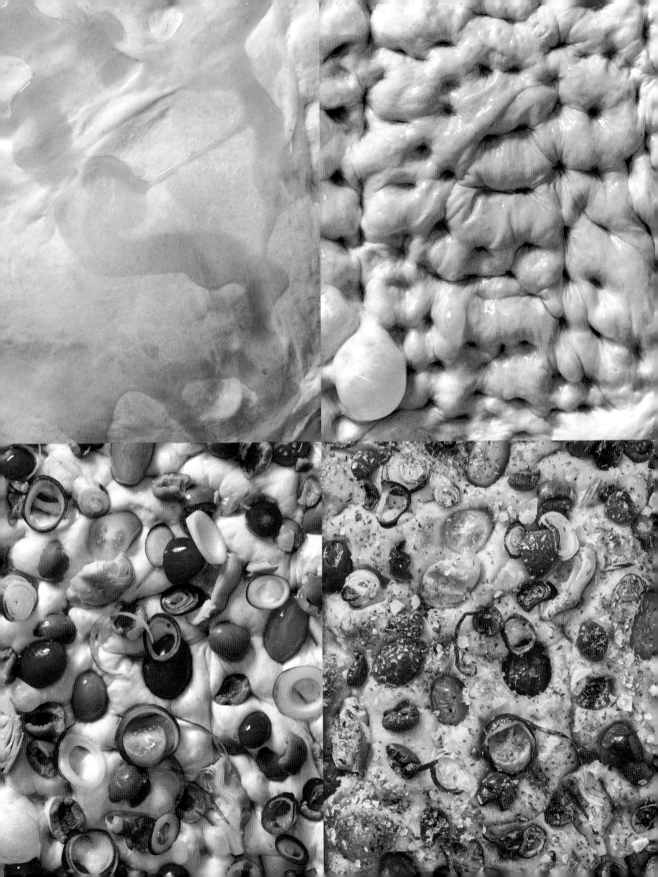

pita

pita In Israel, freshly made pita is available in every corner store. It's honestly next-level incredible. Pita is the perfect side to salads in all forms—you can dip it in tahina or stuff it with leftovers for a satisfying snack. It's worth the effort. **MAKES 10 TO 12 PITA**

FOR THE LEAVEN
10 grams instant yeast
15 grams sugar

FOR THE DOUGH
1 kilogram bread flour
30 grams extra virgin olive oil
25 grams kosher salt

1. MAKE THE LEAVEN: In the bowl of a stand mixer fitted with the paddle attachment, combine the yeast, sugar, and 50 grams lukewarm (110°F to 115°F) water. Let rest for 15 to 20 minutes, until it becomes foamy.

2. MAKE THE DOUGH: Sift the flour into the bowl and pour in 550 grams lukewarm (110°F to 115°F) water. Mix well to combine. Add the olive oil and mix on low speed. Let rest for 10 to 15 minutes.

3. Add the salt and mix on low speed. Let rest again for 10 to 15 minutes.

4. Transfer the dough to a container with a lid and let rise, covered, until at least doubled in size. You can proof it overnight in the refrigerator or at room temperature for 2½ to 3 hours.

5. If you let it rest in the fridge, take the dough out of the fridge about 2 hours before you want to serve. Let it come to room temperature for 1 hour.

6. Divide the dough into ten to twelve equal balls and cover with a kitchen towel. Let rest for 45 minutes to 1 hour.

7. Place a pizza stone in the oven and preheat the oven to 475°F. If you don't have a pizza stone, you can also use a cast-iron skillet on a stove top, but a pizza stone is faster.

8. Working from the center out, roll each ball into a flat circle 5 to 6 inches in diameter.

9. Transfer the circles to the pizza stone and bake for 1½ to 2 minutes, until they puff up. Keep a close eye on the pita so they don't burn. Serve immediately and store any leftovers in a large ziplock bag.

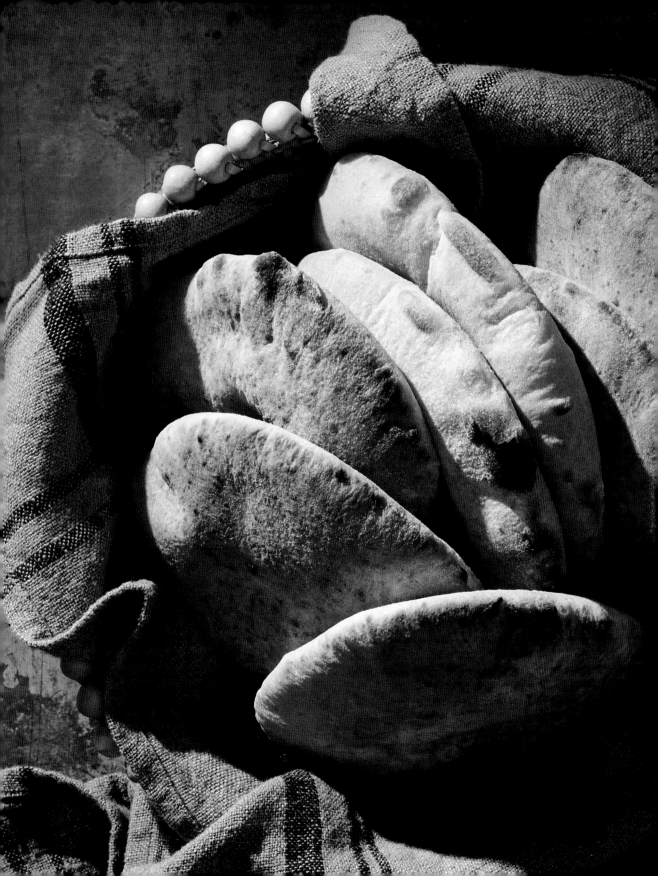

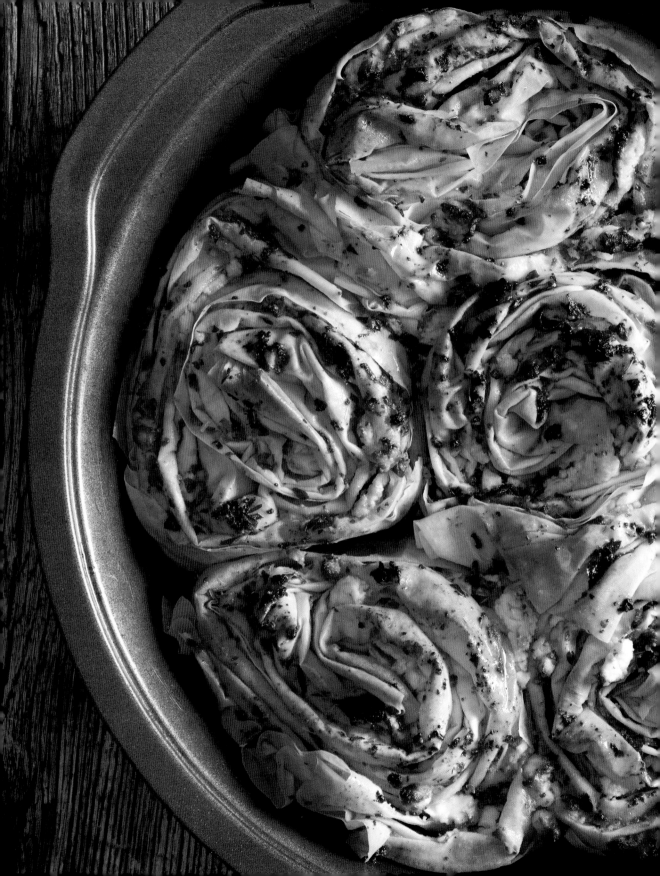

garlicky phyllo bread

This is my one contribution to the bread section, if you can't tell. I had a package of phyllo dough in the freezer that had been there for a while, and I didn't want it to go bad (and I wanted my freezer space back). I brushed on fresh garlic, extra virgin olive oil, and a bunch of herbs and was totally blown away by the results. It's a great recipe for entertaining and is so fun to make. Add your favorite cheeses, olives, caramelized onions, whatever you have that's taking up space. People will be amazed. **SERVES 6 TO 8**

½ cup extra virgin olive oil, plus more for brushing

6 garlic cloves, grated with a Microplane

1 teaspoon fine sea salt

1 tablespoon dried oregano

1 tablespoon garlic powder

3 tablespoons chopped fresh parsley

¼ teaspoon freshly ground black pepper

Juice of ½ lemon (about 1½ tablespoons)

8 to 10 sheets frozen phyllo dough, thawed in the fridge for at least 8 hours

½ cup crumbled feta

1. Preheat the oven to 375°F. Brush a 9-inch pie pan with olive oil (this will also work in a loaf pan if that's all you have).

2. In a small bowl, whisk together the olive oil, grated garlic, salt, oregano, garlic powder, parsley, pepper, and lemon juice.

3. Work with the phyllo two layers at a time. Brush the top layer with the olive oil mixture and sprinkle crumbled feta on top.

4. Scrunch the layers together lengthwise to form a long, accordion-like line. Roll the line of phyllo into a pinwheel and place in the pie pan. Repeat this process until your pie pan is full, around six wheels.

5. Brush the top with the remaining olive oil mixture, making sure to get it in all the nooks and crannies.

6. Bake for 25 to 30 minutes, until the top is golden brown and crispy. Serve immediately.

sourdough starter

A thriving sourdough starter is the foundation for successful bread making. Starters need to be fed every day, which can be a time commitment. To grow your own starter, you can start from scratch using Adi's method below, or you can ask around—many people have some to spare, so heirloom starters aren't hard to find.

how to make a sourdough starter from scratch

305 grams rye flour
105 grams all-purpose flour

1. Add 150 grams room-temperature (around 78°F) filtered water and 100 grams rye flour to a clean jar and stir well with a wooden spoon or rubber spatula to combine. Seal the jar and let sit on the counter for 24 hours.

2. The next day, open the jar and scoop half of the mixture out. (You can throw this away.) Pour in another 150 grams room-temperature water and 100 grams of the rye flour, and mix well with a wooden spoon or rubber spatula so it's all combined. Cover loosely and let sit for another 24 hours.

3. After 24 hours, you should begin to see bubbles form on the sides of the jar. Measure out 75 grams of the starter and throw the rest away. Add the starter to a clean jar and add 75 grams room-temperature water, 35 grams of the rye flour, and 35 grams of the all-purpose flour. Mix everything together well with a wooden spoon or rubber spatula and cover loosely.

4. Repeat step 3 the following day. You should continue to see bubbles form on the side of the jar.

5. The following day, repeat this process. Wrap a rubber band around the jar where the top of the mixture lands so you can see how much it grows.

6. To check if your starter is ready to use, get a bowl of room-temperature water and add 1 tablespoon of the starter. If the starter floats, you're ready to start baking. If it doesn't, continue feeding it following the instructions in step 3 until it's ready.

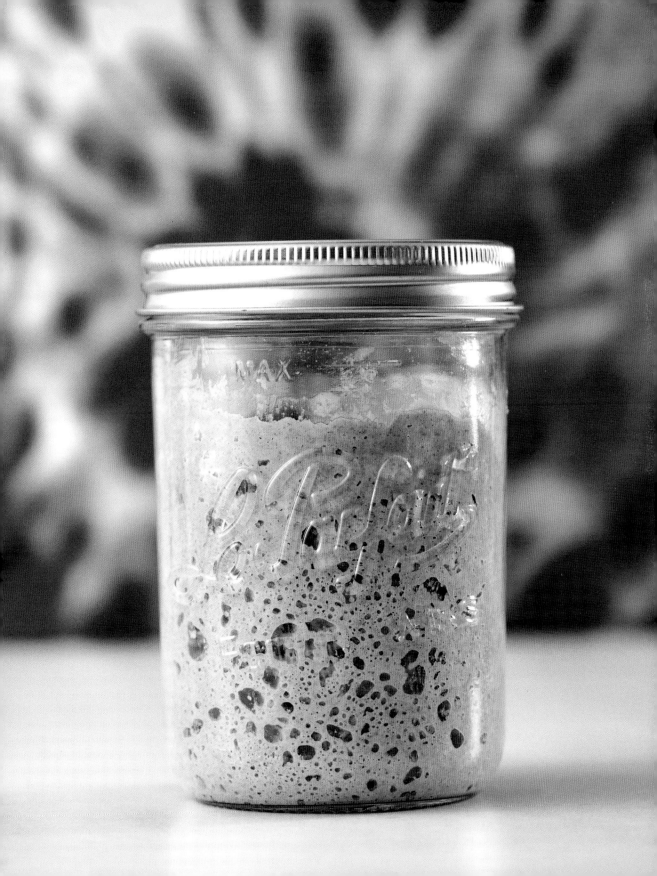

sourdough pizza dough

Good pizza dough is the source of endless creativity. And let me tell you, this dough is good. It creates a crispy base and a soft, pillowy crust that practically melts in your mouth. Just thinking up the ideal toppings could occupy me for hours.

Ever since Adi got his wood-fired outdoor pizza oven, we've loved hosting pizza parties on our roof with friends and neighbors. But if you don't have a pizza oven, you can use this dough recipe in a regular oven or on a grill with equally delicious results. He makes the dough and I beg him to let me decorate it. It does take time—and sought-after refrigerator space—but the result is so worth it. **MAKES ENOUGH FOR FOUR 12-INCH PIZZAS**

FOR THE LEAVEN

5 grams instant yeast

35 grams active sourdough starter (see page 198)

15 grams sugar

FOR THE DOUGH

550 grams bread flour, plus more for dusting

30 grams extra virgin olive oil

10 grams kosher salt

Cornmeal, for dusting

1. MAKE THE LEAVEN: In the bowl of a stand mixer fitted with the paddle attachment, combine the yeast, starter, sugar, and 50 grams lukewarm (110°F to 115°F) water. Let rest for 15 to 20 minutes, until foamy.

2. MAKE THE DOUGH: Add 370 grams lukewarm (110°F to 115°F) water to the bowl and sift in the bread flour in three parts. Mix well to combine on low to medium speed after each addition and let it rest for 2 minutes in between so the gluten relaxes. Add the olive oil and mix on low speed. Let rest for another 10 to 15 minutes, until the dough is stretchy enough to pull without breaking.

3. Finally, add the salt and mix on low speed until it's fully incorporated. Let rest for 10 to 15 minutes, until the dough is stretchy enough to pull without breaking.

4. Transfer the dough to a container with a lid. Cover and let rest for 10 to 15 minutes.

5. Remove the cover and stretch and fold the dough. Let rest for another 10 to 15 minutes, then repeat the stretch-and-fold process two more times.

6. After the last round of stretching, cover the dough and let it rise until at least doubled in size, about 3 hours. For best flavor, place the dough in the fridge overnight, then let it come to room temperature by removing the dough from the fridge 2 hours before you want to serve and letting it sit at room temperature for 1 hour.

7. Divide the dough into four equal balls. Let rest for 45 minutes to 1 hour.

if you're using an oven

1. I recommend using a pizza stone. We use a ceramic one; they typically come in a few different sizes, but 14 to 16 inches diameter should suffice for daily use. Preheat the oven to 500°F and heat the stone in the oven for at least 45 minutes before baking the pizza so the stone doesn't crack.

2. Dust a flat surface with cornmeal and turn the dough out. Flatten each dough ball into a 10- to 12-inch round, curving your hands as you go to make a slight crust.

3. Add your favorite toppings to the dough and carefully transfer to the pizza stone.

4. Lower the oven temperature to 475°F and bake for 3 to 5 minutes, until the pizza crust is golden brown.

if you're using a grill

1. Place a pizza stone on the grill and preheat to high (minimum 450°F).

2. Dust a flat surface with cornmeal and turn the dough out. Flatten each dough ball into a 10- to 12-inch round, curving your hands as you go to make a slight crust. Place the dough on the hottest part of the stone.

3. Close the grill and wait 30 seconds to 1 minute.

4. Flip the dough and close the grill for another 30 seconds.

5. Carefully remove the pizza dough and add your toppings (see the following recipes). If using cheese, place the pizza back on the grill and let your cheese melt. Remove from the grill and enjoy immediately.

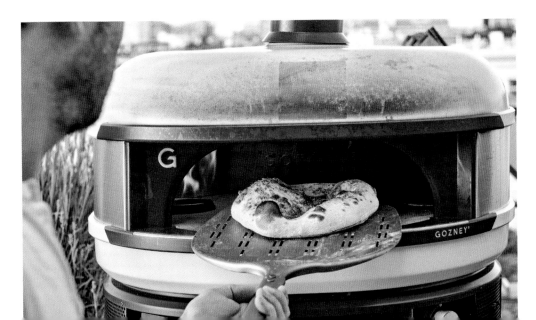

heirloom tomato pizza

When you're using fresh dough, it only makes sense to highlight it with the freshest ingredients. Whenever I'm in charge of decorating the pizzas, I make this. It lets all the juiciest local farm stand tomatoes shine alongside fresh garlic, extra virgin olive oil, and a touch of Parmesan. So simple, but so mind-blowingly good. **MAKES TWO 12-INCH PIZZAS**

Cornmeal, for dusting

2 sourdough pizza dough balls (see page 200)

2 large heirloom tomatoes

Fine sea salt

6 garlic cloves, grated with a Microplane

⅔ cup extra virgin olive oil

2 cups grated Parmesan

2 cups arugula

Juice of 1 lemon (about 3 tablespoons)

Freshly ground black pepper

1. Preheat the oven to 500°F and place a pizza stone inside for at least 45 minutes before baking the pizza so it doesn't crack.

2. Dust a flat surface with cornmeal and turn the dough out. Flatten each dough ball into a 12-inch round, curving your hands as you go to make a slight crust.

3. Cut the tomatoes into ¼-inch slices and pat dry with a paper towel. Salt the slices and pat dry again.

4. In a small bowl, whisk together the garlic and ⅓ cup of the olive oil.

5. Sprinkle ½ cup of the Parmesan across each dough round.

6. Neatly cover the cheese with the tomato slices.

7. Brush the tomatoes with the garlic–olive oil mixture. Use any remaining oil to brush the crusts.

8. Sprinkle the remaining 1 cup Parmesan over the tomatoes.

9. Carefully place one of the pizzas on the pizza stone. Lower the oven temperature to 475°F and bake for 3 to 5 minutes, until the crust is golden brown. Repeat with the remaining pizza.

10. In a medium bowl, toss together the arugula with the remaining ⅓ cup olive oil and lemon juice. Season with salt and pepper to taste.

11. Top the pizzas with the dressed arugula. Serve immediately. Store any leftovers in an airtight container in the fridge for up to 2 days.

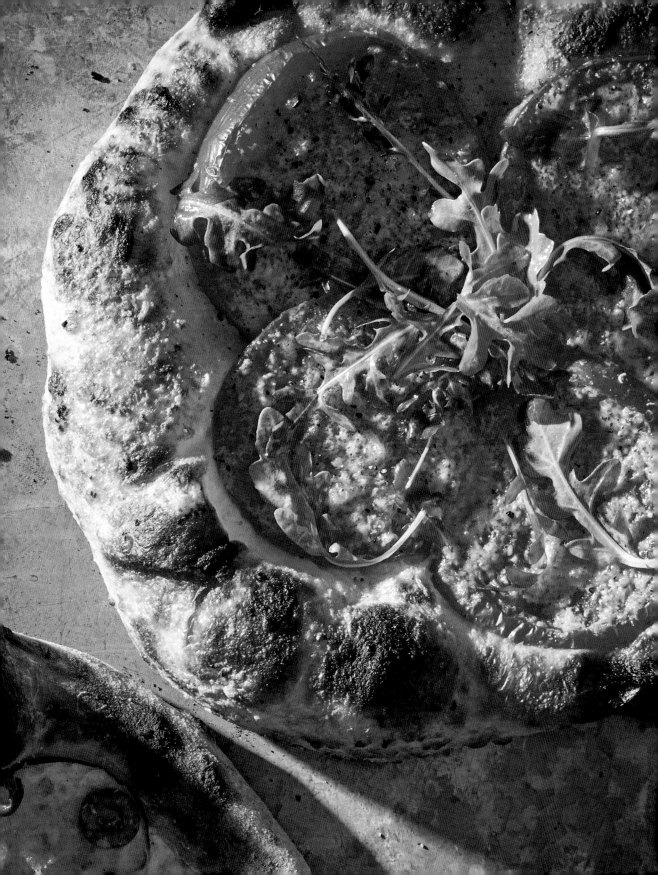

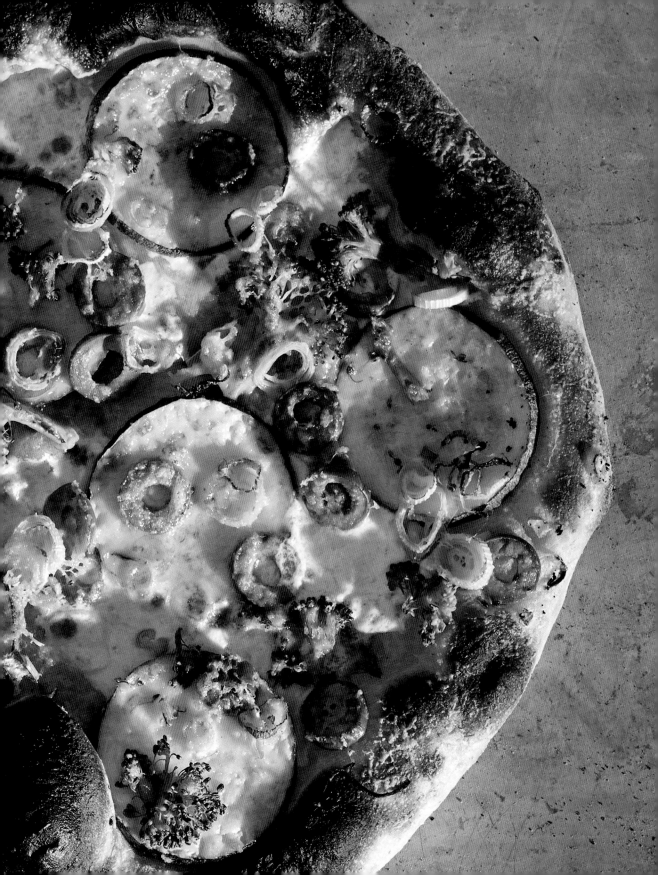

green veggie pizza

When you eat as much pizza as we do, you can get tired of eating the same old cheese variety. (That is, unless you're my kids.) To vary our toppings, I let my produce drawer provide inspiration, and some days it just works. This is one of my favorites. The combination of juicy zucchini, salty olives, and crunchy broccoli that gets just a little bit charred in the oven is one of the most delectable, enjoyable meals I eat on any given week. The veggies shine through layers of creamy, melted cheese and give you a taste of just about everything good in the world.

MAKES TWO 12-INCH PIZZAS

Cornmeal, for dusting

2 sourdough pizza dough balls (see page 200)

½ cup sliced Castelvetrano olives

2 zucchini, cut into ¼-inch discs

1 head broccoli, cut into small florets

4 scallions, trimmed, white and light green parts thinly sliced (about ½ cup)

1 cup sliced fresh mozzarella

Freshly grated Parmesan, to garnish

1. Preheat the oven to 500°F and place a pizza stone inside for at least 45 minutes before baking the bread so it doesn't crack.

2. Dust a flat surface with cornmeal and turn the dough out. Flatten each dough ball into a 12-inch round, curving your hands as you go to make a slight crust.

3. Top the crust with the olives, then zucchini, broccoli, scallions, mozzarella, and Parmesan.

4. Carefully place one pizza on the pizza stone. Lower the oven temperature to 475°F and bake for 3 to 5 minutes, until the crust is golden brown. Transfer the pizza to a wire rack and repeat with the remaining pizza. Serve immediately. Store any leftovers in the fridge in an airtight container for up to 2 days.

za'atar bread

We always have za'atar from the Israeli market in our pantry. It's herby and bright, with a hint of nuttiness from the sesame seeds. If we ever have pizza dough on hand, we make this bread to eat with our meal and scoop up all the confetti-size bites of veggies. It's simple but adds just the right amount of flavor to round out any meal. **MAKES TWO 12-INCH PIZZAS**

Cornmeal, for dusting

2 sourdough pizza dough balls (see page 200)

¼ cup extra virgin olive oil

2 teaspoons za'atar

1 teaspoon fine sea salt

2 tablespoons chopped fresh chives

2 tablespoons chopped fresh parsley

1 to 2 scallions, trimmed, light green and white parts thinly sliced (about 2 tablespoons)

1. Preheat the oven to 500°F and place a pizza stone inside for at least 45 minutes before baking the bread so it doesn't crack.

2. Dust a flat surface with cornmeal and turn the dough out. Flatten each dough ball into a 12-inch round, curving your hands as you go to make a slight crust.

3. In a small bowl, whisk together the olive oil, za'atar, salt, chives, and parsley.

4. Spread the oil mixture over the dough.

5. Carefully place one of the breads on the pizza stone. Lower the oven temperature to 475°F and bake for 3 to 5 minutes, until the crust is golden brown. Transfer the hot bread to a wire rack and repeat with the remaining breads.

6. Garnish with the scallions and serve immediately. Store any leftovers in the fridge in an airtight container for up to 2 days.

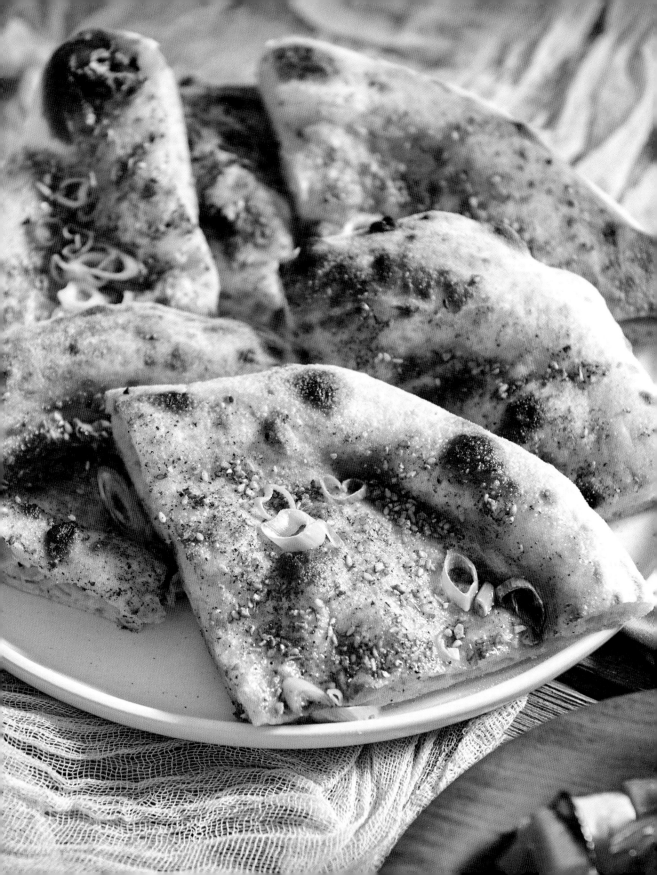

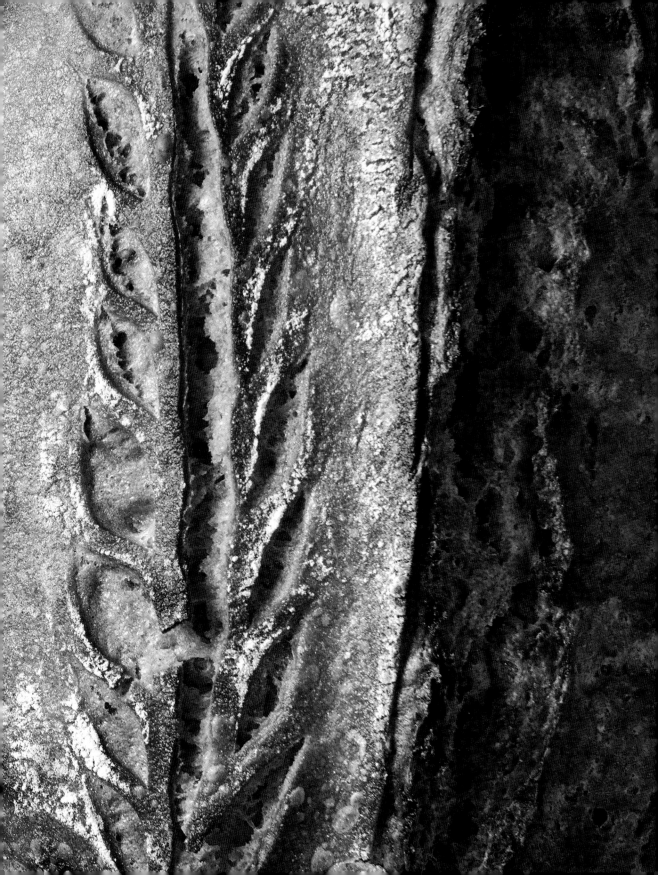

sourdough loaf

For Adi's birthday in 2020, I ordered bread for him from Poilâne—Paris's renowned sourdough bakery—plus everything else he needed to make sourdough, which he seemed to like at the time but didn't really dive into. Three weeks later, the world shut down and everyone went into lockdown as a result of COVID-19. He spent the whole pandemic mastering his sourdough recipe and nurturing a homemade starter, even after a few mishaps (including once when I accidentally baked it). Fresh sourdough bread is a labor of love, but my girls and I love it and are so lucky to have someone to make it for us. You'll never eat a better meal than a crispy grilled cheese made with butter and fresh sourdough, I promise. **MAKES 2 LOAVES**

FOR THE LEAVEN

50 grams organic bread flour

50 grams T85 flour (see page 192)

100 grams active sourdough starter (see page 198)

FOR THE DOUGH

300 grams einkorn flour

450 grams organic bread flour

250 grams T70 flour (see page 192)

25 grams fine sea salt

Rice flour, for dusting

Make the leaven the night before making the dough. For a 100 percent hydrated active starter fed at 4 p.m., make the leaven around 10 p.m.

1. MAKE THE LEAVEN: In a small bowl, mix together the bread flour, T85 flour, sourdough starter, and 100 grams room-temperature water. Cover and let rest overnight at room temperature.

2. MAKE THE DOUGH: In a large bowl, combine the einkorn flour, bread flour, T70 flour, and 750 grams room-temperature water. Mix lightly by hand and let the dough rest, covered, for 30 to 60 minutes so the flour can hydrate.

3. Add 165 grams of the leaven to the dough and mix vigorously with your hands. Cover with a kitchen towel and let rest for 15 minutes, then mix in the salt with your hands. Once everything is incorporated, begin to stretch and fold the dough by pulling each edge up in quarters and folding from 2 o'clock to 7 o'clock. Repeat this process across the whole bowl.

4. Scrape down the sides of the bowl, cover, and let rest for 15 minutes.

(continued)

5. Uncover the dough and repeat the stretch-and-fold process for 1 minute. Cover and let rest for another 15 minutes.

6. Repeat the process once more and let rest for 15 minutes more.

7. After 15 minutes, fold the dough over itself and transfer it to a clean bowl. Let sit, covered, for at least 6 hours to overnight in a warm place.

8. Turn the dough out on a lightly floured surface and divide into two equal pieces. Roughly shape the dough with a bench scraper based on the proofing baskets you're planning to use. Let rest uncovered for 40 minutes so the crust can develop.

9. Flour the proofing baskets or a towel with rice flour. Now shape the dough. Dust a flat surface with rice flour as well and turn the dough upside down onto it and stretch the dough lightly. Fold the bottom into the middle, then fold the top into the middle over it like an envelope. Turn the dough lengthwise and roll it toward you. Tuck the ends under and place seam side up in the proofing basket or a bowl lined with the towel. Pinch the edges and pull them into the center so the dough is taut. Repeat with the second loaf.

10. Let proof overnight or for at least 12 hours, covered, in the refrigerator.

11. In the morning, place a Dutch oven in the oven and preheat to 500°F.

12. Once the oven is preheated, carefully turn the dough out of the proofing basket onto a piece of parchment paper. Score a curved line across the top of the dough with a lame or sharp paring knife.

13. Remove the Dutch oven from the hot oven and lift the parchment paper and dough into the pot. Add two or three ice cubes to create a steam puff (it will prevent the crust from forming too fast). Cover the Dutch oven with its lid, lower the oven temperature to 475°F, and bake the bread for 20 minutes.

14. Lower the temperature to 450°F. Remove the lid of the Dutch oven and bake for another 25 minutes, until the top of the loaf is dark golden brown. Remove the loaf from the Dutch oven and repeat with the second loaf.

15. Let cool completely on a wire rack before cutting. Store any leftovers in a large ziplock bag or your preferred method of bread storage for up to 4 days.

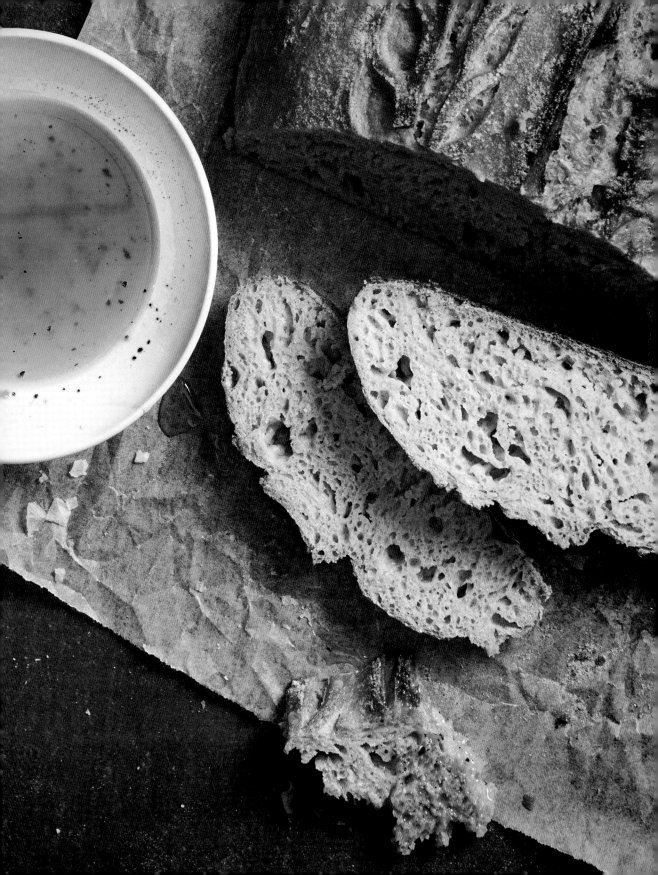

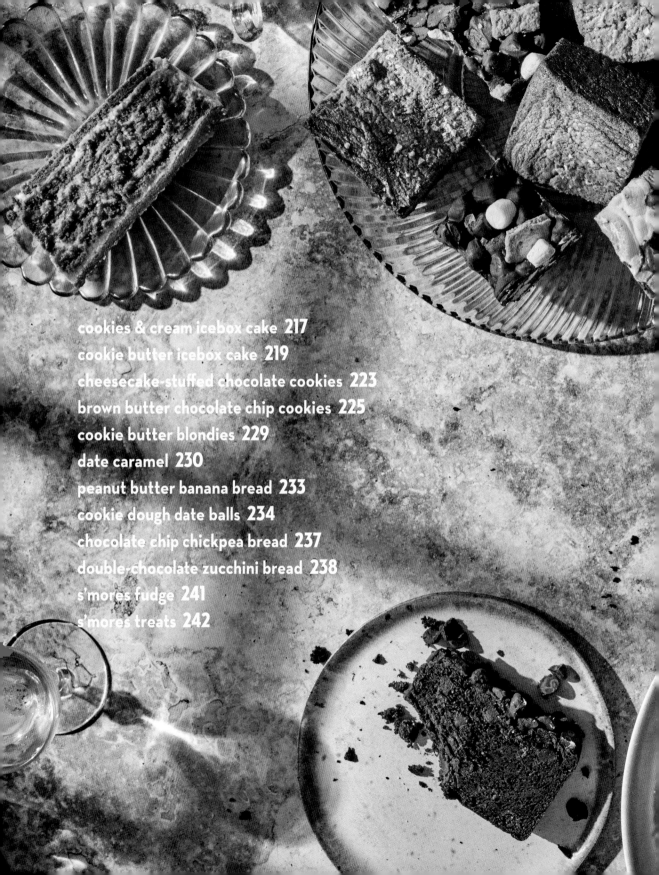

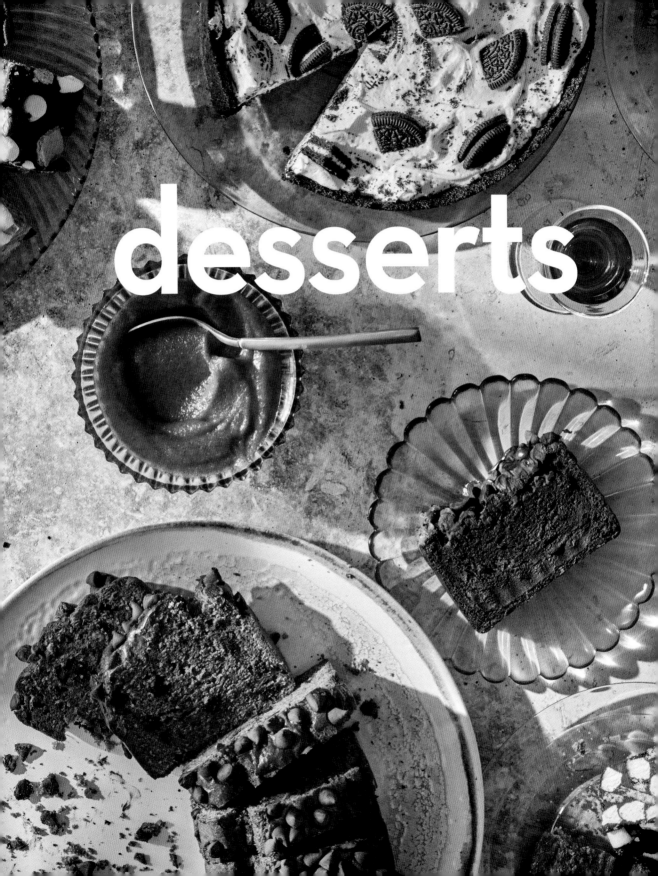

desserts

I'm a dessert person—I crave a bite of something sweet at the end of every meal. At Baked by Melissa, whenever I'm developing a new flavor, my goal is to create the perfect combination of flavors and textures all in one bite. Many of these cupcake flavors are inspired by desserts I loved as a kid, and all of them are meant to make people happy. The desserts I make at home are also inspired by childhood favorites, sometimes with a twist. You'll often find me in the kitchen at night dreaming up ways to make something delicious that satisfies my kids and my sweet tooth. Most of the time it involves chocolate, and many times it allows little fingers to help.

There are a lot of dessert recipes in my repertoire, many of which you can find in my dessert-focused book, *Cakes by Melissa,* but I handpicked the recipes in this book because they're my absolute favorites. They're the ones that make their way into our weekly schedule, that impress guests, and that I always want more of. Make them with your kids, pass them down, and claim them as your own—you have my permission. As long as you're making and enjoying them, I'll be happy.

"I crave a bite of something sweet at the end of every meal."

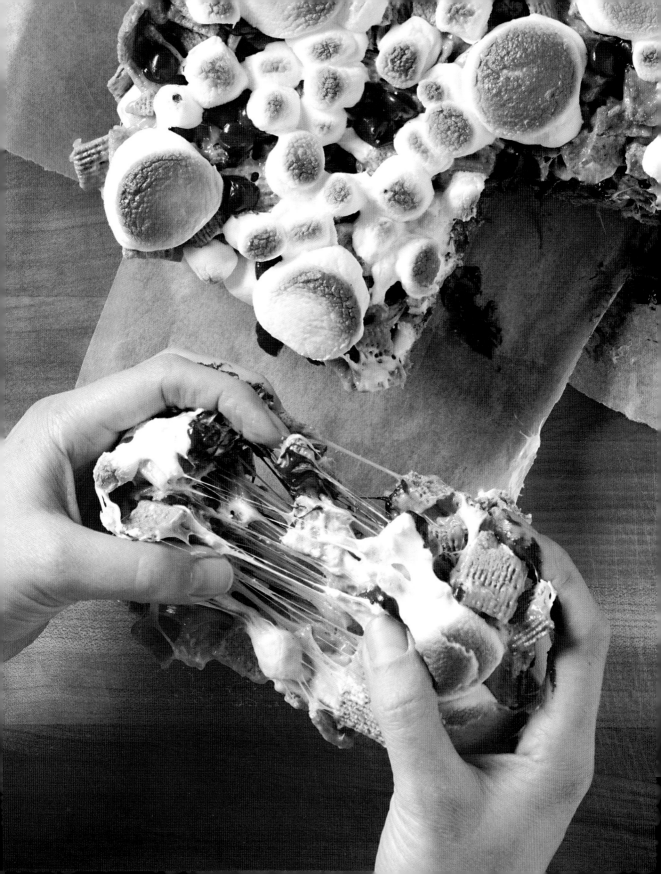

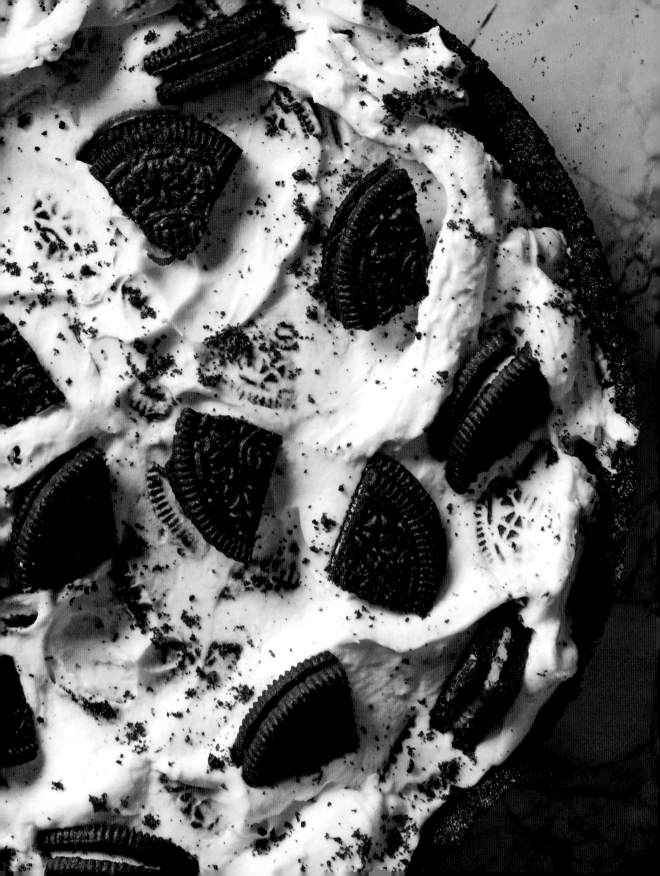

cookies & cream icebox cake

I love icebox cakes because they give you the chance to be creative and have fun while making something absolutely mouthwatering. The best cookies-and-cream desserts use the entire Oreo, not just the cookies, so I did just that. Each and every bite tastes like the perfect combo of cookies and cream, brightened with a touch of lemon. **SERVES 8**

Two 14.3-ounce packages Oreos

8 tablespoons (1 stick) unsalted butter, melted

2 cups cold heavy cream

8 ounces (1 block) cream cheese, at room temperature

½ cup sugar

1 teaspoon vanilla extract

½ teaspoon fine sea salt

Juice of ½ lemon (about 1½ tablespoons)

½ teaspoon lemon zest

1. Put one package of the Oreos into a food processor or blender and process until you have a sandy texture. Add the melted butter. Stir together until a doughy consistency forms.

2. Press your crust evenly along the bottom and up the sides of a 9-inch pie pan using the bottom of a glass. Don't worry about greasing the pan because there's butter in the crust. Be patient with this step! An even crust will look really beautiful, so make sure to spend those few extra minutes.

3. Remove two sleeves from the second package Oreos. Chop the cookies coarsely into quarters, or whatever size cookie chunks you like best.

4. Pour the heavy cream into a stand mixer fitted with the whisk attachment and whip on high speed until it has a whipped cream consistency, 3 to 5 minutes. Swap out the whisk for a paddle attachment and add the softened cream cheese. Beat on medium-low speed until just combined.

5. Add the sugar, vanilla, salt, lemon juice, and lemon zest. Mix until combined. Fold the Oreo chunks into the whipped cream and pour the mixture into the crust.

6. Decorate the top of the cake with any remaining whole Oreos left in the pack.

7. Cover the cake and refrigerate for at least 24 hours, or up to 3 days, to soften the cookies completely.

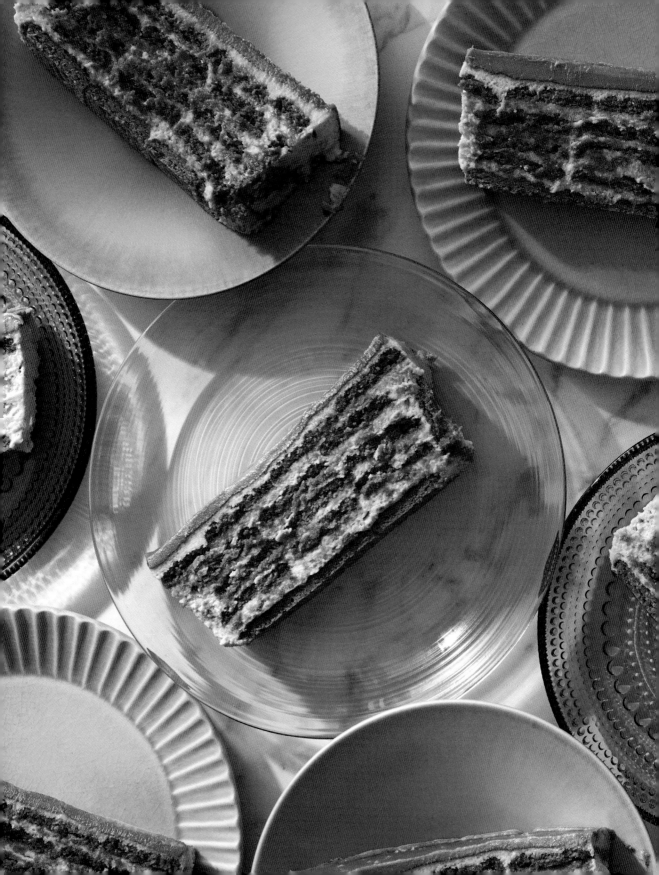

cookie butter icebox cake

I've used Biscoff spread—aka cookie butter—as an ingredient at every possible opportunity since I first tried the creamy, dreamy, liquid graham-cracker-esque spread many years ago at the Food & Wine Classic. At least once a year, we create a Biscoff-inspired flavor for Baked by Melissa, whether it's overstuffed or topped with the dreamy spread (or both!). I first made this cake for my best friend Bari's son's second birthday, and it was, simply, the best dessert ever. It has the texture of an icebox cake; the sweet, spiced flavor of Biscoff; and incredible balance from a sprinkle of flaky salt. It's absolutely next level, and my girls love helping me arrange the cookies for each layer. **SERVES 8**

2 cups cold heavy cream

4 ounces (½ block) cream cheese, at room temperature

1 cup Biscoff cookie butter

1 teaspoon vanilla extract

1 teaspoon lemon juice

2 tablespoons sugar

½ teaspoon fine sea salt

Two 8.8-ounce sleeves Biscoff cookies

Flaky sea salt, to garnish

1. Pour the heavy cream into the bowl of a stand mixer fitted with the whisk attachment and whip on high speed until it has a whipped cream consistency, 3 to 5 minutes. Stir in the cream cheese.

2. Stir in ½ cup of the cookie butter. Add the vanilla and lemon juice and stir. Add the sugar and salt and mix until just combined.

3. Line a 1-pound loaf pan with parchment paper, leaving enough paper on each side to use as a tab to lift the icebox cake out. It helps to hold the paper down with metal binder clips.

4. Add a layer of the Biscoff cookies to the bottom of the loaf pan, with the logo facing up.

5. Spread a layer of the whipped cream mixture over the cookies. Cover with another layer of cookies.

6. Repeat this process of layering cookies and whipped cream until the pan is full, ending with a layer of cookies.

(continued)

7. In a small microwave-safe bowl, microwave the remaining ½ cup cookie butter in 15-second increments until melted. Pour the warm cookie butter over the cookies to create a seal.

8. Sprinkle with flaky sea salt and cover. Refrigerate for at least 24 hours, or up to 3 days, to soften the cookies completely. Carefully lift the cake out of the pan (you may need to run a knife along the edges) and serve in slices.

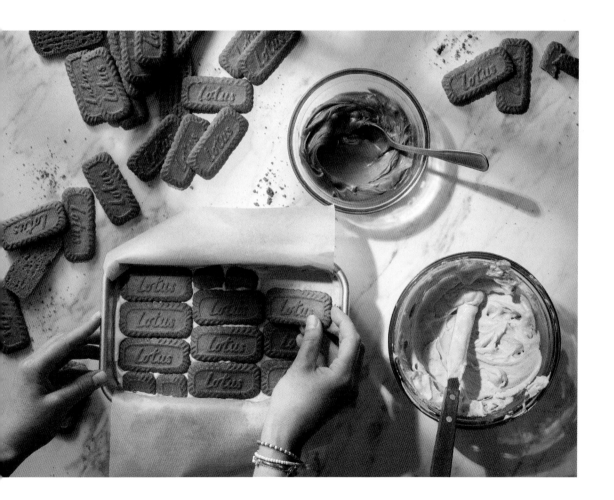

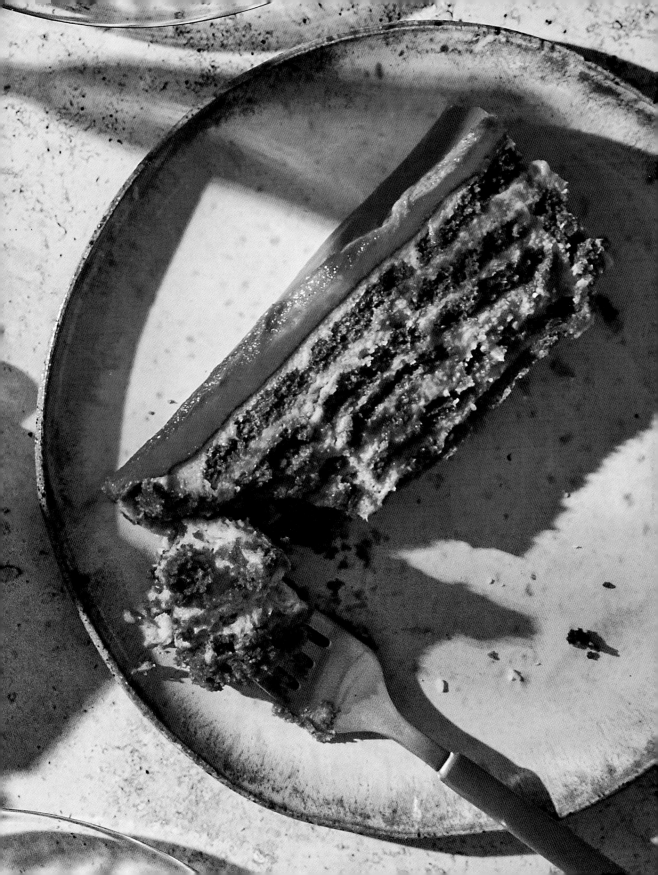

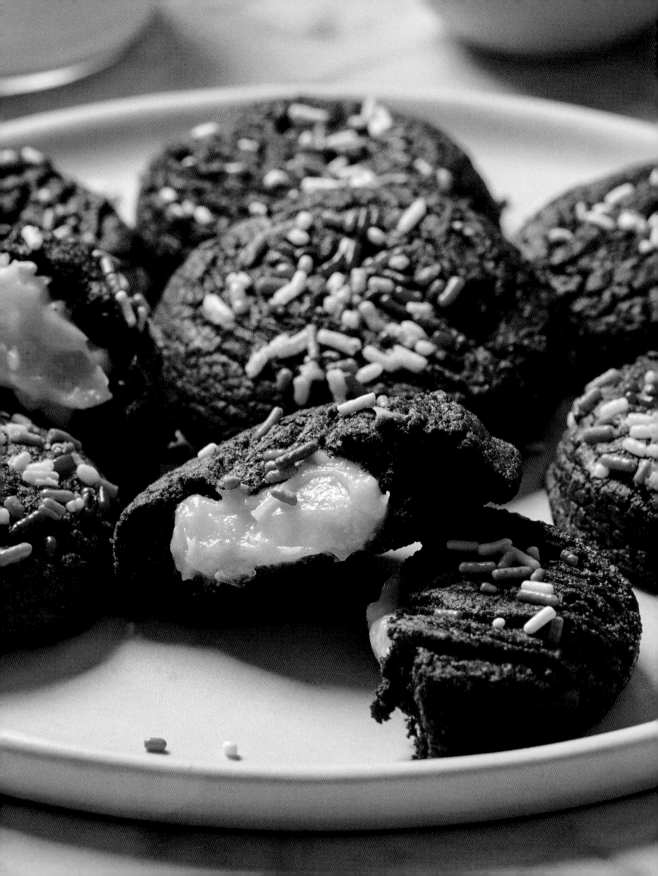

cheesecake-stuffed chocolate cookies

Whether you're making a salad dressing or a chocolate layer cake, once you get the basics down, you have so much freedom to experiment and create based on what you love. And I love Oreos, so finding new ways to include them in desserts is a dream come true. Truthfully, when I first made this, I wasn't sure these cookies were going to work, but I am so happy they did. They're sort of like soft-baked Oreos, filled with a delicious cheesecake stuffing. But don't limit yourself to cheesecake stuffing—these cookies can be filled with peanut butter, cookie butter, leftover Halloween candy, anything you have. **MAKES 16 COOKIES**

FOR THE CHEESECAKE FILLING

16 ounces (2 blocks) cream cheese, at room temperature

1 teaspoon vanilla extract

¼ cup plus 1 tablespoon sugar

Juice of ½ lemon (about 1½ tablespoons)

Pinch of fine sea salt

½ cup rainbow sprinkles, plus more for decorating

FOR THE CHOCOLATE COOKIE DOUGH

24 Oreo cookies

4 tablespoons (½ stick) unsalted butter, at room temperature

1 large egg, at room temperature

¼ cup sugar

½ teaspoon baking powder

½ cup plus 1 tablespoon all-purpose flour

1. Line a baking sheet with parchment paper.

2. MAKE THE CHEESECAKE FILLING: In a stand mixer fitted with the paddle attachment, combine the cream cheese, vanilla, and sugar. Mix on high until fluffy, 3 to 5 minutes.

3. Add the lemon juice and salt and mix to combine. Fold in the sprinkles.

4. Portion out the cheesecake filling in 1-tablespoon scoops and place them on the baking sheet. Freeze for 2 hours or until solid.

5. MAKE THE COOKIE DOUGH: Add the Oreos to a blender or food processor and process until the mixture reaches a sand-like consistency.

6. Transfer the Oreo crumbs into the bowl of a stand mixer fitted with the paddle attachment. Add the butter, egg, sugar, and baking powder. Mix on medium speed until combined. With the mixer on low, slowly add in the flour until it begins to form a dough.

(continued)

7. Preheat the oven to 350°F and line a baking sheet with parchment paper. Remove the cheesecake filling from the freezer.

8. Portion the cookie dough using a 1-inch scoop. Press a piece of cheesecake filling into the dough and cover with cookie dough.

9. Dip the cookie in rainbow sprinkles.

10. Place the cookies 1 inch apart on the prepared baking sheet. Depending on the size of your pan, you may need to bake these in two or three batches. Bake the cookies for 12 minutes, until the edges are dry and the middle looks soft and mostly set. Immediately after removing the cookies from the oven, swirl a wide-mouth glass around the cookies to create perfect circles. Store the cookies in an airtight container for up to 5 days.

brown butter chocolate chip cookies

Once you've made these cookies, you'll never want to make any other chocolate chip cookie again. They're the best. The brown butter elevates the flavor and texture of the cookies, giving them a rich nuttiness that's to die for.

This recipe includes a few of my tricks for taking your cookie game to the next level. Use a scoop to measure out the dough, place chocolate chips on top of the dough before you bake, and underbake for just a minute or two for gooey results. A sprinkle of flaky sea salt at the end really makes the chocolate pop. Go make these now and pass down this recipe for generations. **MAKES 16 COOKIES**

1 cup (2 sticks) unsalted butter
¾ cup packed light brown sugar
¾ cup granulated sugar
2 large eggs, at room temperature
1 teaspoon vanilla extract
2¼ cups all-purpose flour
1 teaspoon baking soda
1 teaspoon fine sea salt
1¼ cups chocolate chips
Flaky sea salt

1. Start by browning your butter. Heat a saucepan over medium heat and add the butter. As the butter melts, whisk frequently. After a few minutes, it should begin to foam, and you'll notice brown specks at the bottom of the pan. Continue whisking. Don't walk away from the stove during this process—brown butter quickly goes from browned to burnt, so keep an eye on it. When the butter reaches a caramel color with brown specks at the bottom, remove it from the heat immediately. It should have a nutty aroma. Pour the butter into a heat-safe bowl, scraping all the brown bits in. Let it cool to room temperature.

2. Preheat the oven to 375°F and line a baking sheet with parchment paper.

3. Add the cooled brown butter, brown sugar, and granulated sugar to the bowl of a stand mixer fitted with the paddle attachment. Beat on high until light and fluffy, 3 to 5 minutes.

4. Add the eggs to the mixer one at a time, combining well after each addition. Stir in the vanilla.

(continued)

5. With the mixer on low, add the flour, baking soda, and salt to the bowl. Mix until just combined, then fold in 1 cup of the chocolate chips.

6. Using a 1-inch scoop, portion out the dough on the cookie sheet, about 1 inch apart. You may need to bake two or three batches depending on the size of your baking sheet.

7. Press the remaining ¼ cup chocolate chips into the tops of the dough balls.

8. Bake for 11 to 12 minutes, until the cookies are golden around the edges and mostly set in the middle. As soon as you remove them from the oven, swirl a wide-mouth glass around the cookies to create perfect circles.

9. Sprinkle with flaky sea salt and let the cookies cool completely on a wire rack. Store any leftovers in an airtight container for 3 to 5 days.

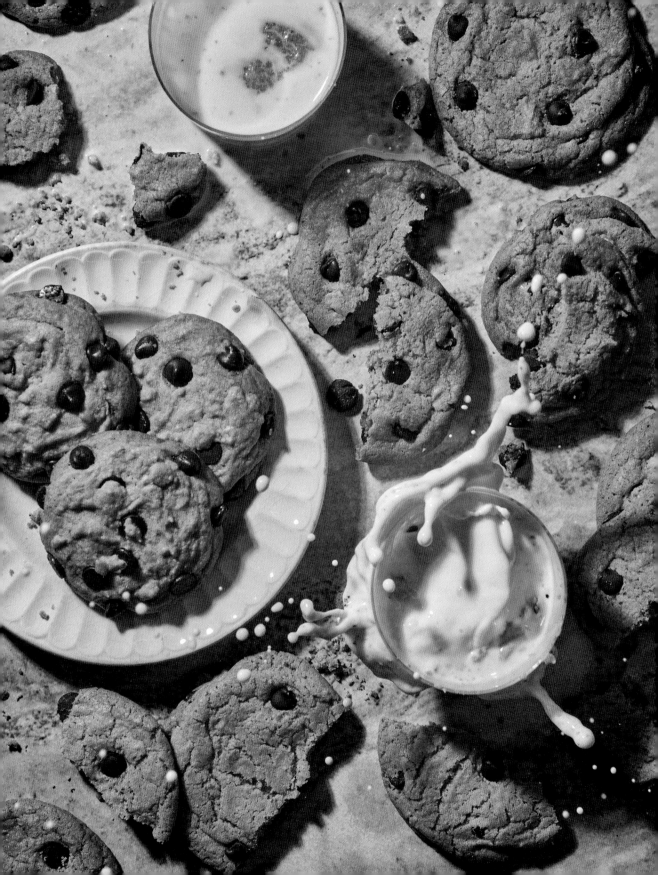

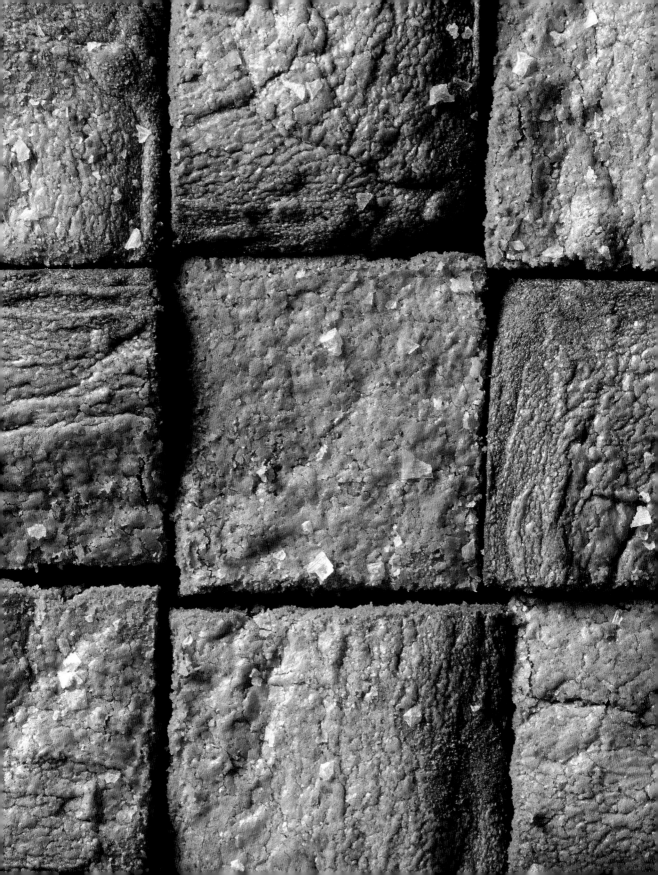

cookie butter blondies

If you thought you liked brownies, these will give them a run for their money. The cookie butter base and cookie crumbs result in a rich, fudgy texture. I highly recommend that you use Biscoff for these, but any cookie butter would work. But the flaky sea salt at the end? Not optional. **MAKES 16 BLONDIES**

¾ cup (1½ sticks) unsalted butter, softened

1 cup packed light brown sugar

4 large eggs, at room temperature

2 teaspoons vanilla paste or extract

20 Biscoff cookies, crushed

Two 14.1-ounce jars Biscoff cookie butter

⅔ cup all-purpose flour

2 teaspoons fine sea salt

1 teaspoon baking powder

Flaky sea salt, to garnish

1. Preheat the oven to 325°F and line a 9-inch square metal baking pan with parchment paper.

2. In the bowl of a stand mixer fitted with the paddle attachment, cream the butter and sugar on high speed until light and fluffy, about 3 minutes. Scrape down the sides of the mixer bowl. Add the eggs one at a time, mixing well after each addition and scraping down the sides of the bowl as you go. Stir in the vanilla, then the crushed cookies and cookie butter.

3. In a large bowl, combine the flour, salt, and baking powder.

4. Add the dry mixture slowly to the stand mixer just until no streaks remain, being careful not to overmix.

5. Pour the batter into the prepared pan. Bake for about 60 minutes, until golden. Garnish with flaky sea salt. Store leftovers in an airtight container for up to 3 days.

date caramel

I have a confession: This isn't actually caramel, but you could probably fool a lot of people with it. The reason I call it caramel is because it has the smooth, creamy texture of caramel that I love and lots of natural sweetness. To make it, you have to soften the dates with boiling water, then pulse them into a spread. I tried to make this many, many times before I did it successfully, and am so happy to share the delicious results with you. I use this caramel to make my Cookie Dough Date Balls (page 234), in place of dates and maple syrup in the Double-Chocolate Zucchini Bread (page 238), or even to top pancakes. Keep a jar of this on hand and you'll always have a way to satisfy your sweet tooth. **MAKES 2 CUPS**

15 Medjool dates, pitted

½ cup organic full-fat coconut cream (make sure to include the solid part from the top of the can)

2 teaspoons vanilla paste or extract

½ teaspoon fine sea salt

1. Place the dates in a small bowl and cover with boiling water for 15 minutes to soften.

2. Transfer the soaked dates to a blender with ¼ cup of the water from the bowl and the coconut cream. Blend until smooth and pour into a 24-ounce jar.

3. Add the vanilla and salt. Mix in the jar and cool completely. Store covered in the refrigerator for up to 2 weeks.

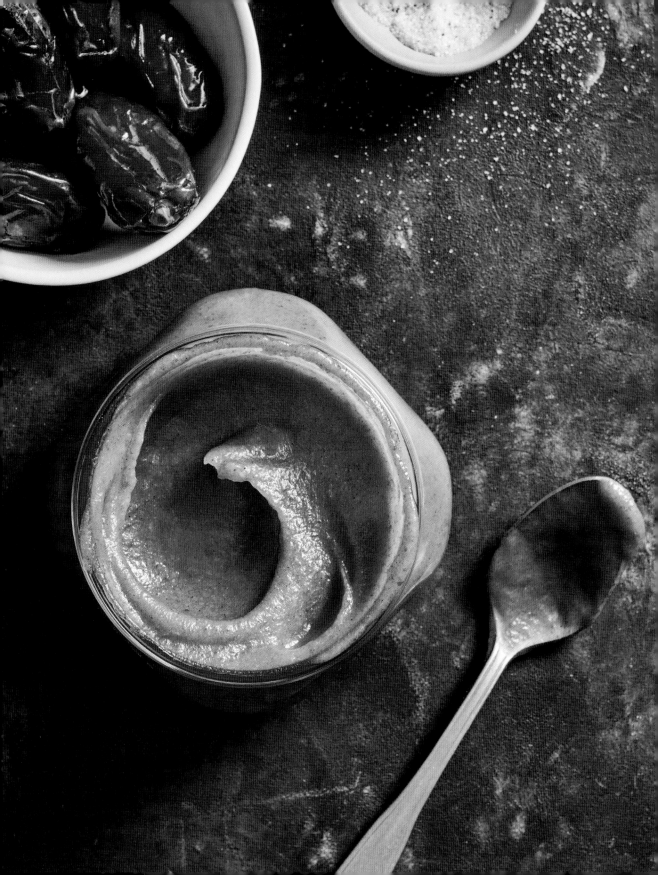

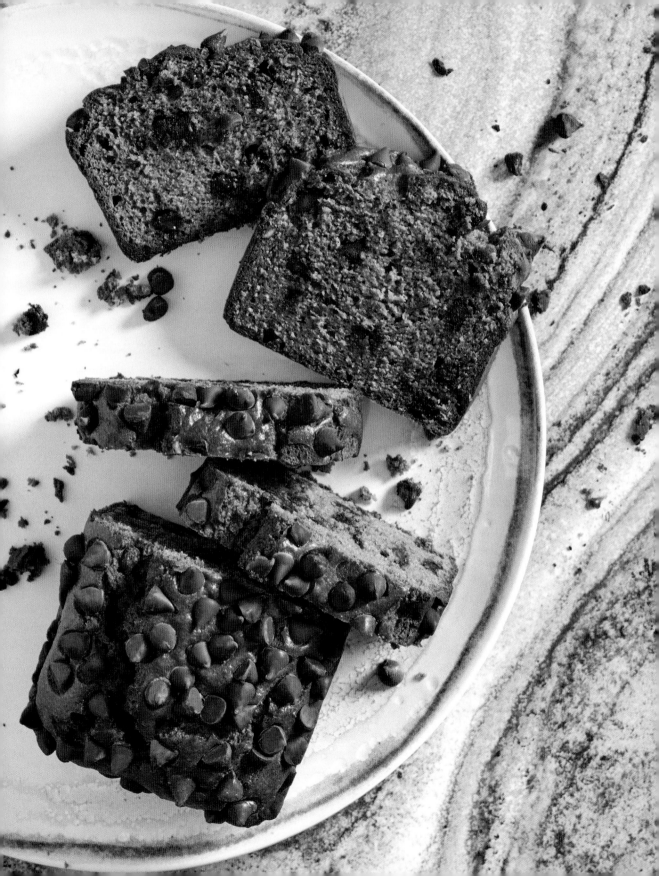

peanut butter banana bread

As a working mom, there are few desserts I like more than those that can be made in a blender. The first time I made this banana bread, I just threw nutrient-rich ingredients that I found in my kitchen into a blender to make the batter. I make it as a loaf, but you can use the same batter for muffins; just reduce the bake time and take them out of the oven when the tops are golden brown. It's hard to go wrong when you combine peanut butter, chocolate chips, and bananas—my kids love it, I love it, and it could easily work for dessert or breakfast.

MAKES 1 LOAF

3 medium ripe or overripe bananas

1½ teaspoons vanilla extract

3 large eggs, at room temperature

⅓ cup maple syrup

½ teaspoon fine sea salt

1 cup creamy peanut butter (or any nut butter)

5 Brazil nuts (optional)

⅓ cup tahina

1 teaspoon baking powder

½ teaspoon baking soda

1 cup rolled oats

1 cup chocolate chips

1. Preheat the oven to 350°F and line the bottom and sides of a 1-pound loaf pan with parchment paper. Leave about 2 inches of parchment paper hanging over the sides to help you pull the bread out later.

2. Add the bananas, vanilla, eggs, maple syrup, salt, peanut butter, Brazil nuts, if using, tahina, baking powder, baking soda, and oats to a high-powered blender. Blend on high until smooth.

3. Fold in ½ cup of the chocolate chips and pour into the prepared loaf pan. Top with the remaining ½ cup chocolate chips.

4. Bake for 35 to 40 minutes, until the top is golden brown. Remove the bread from the pan using the parchment paper tabs and cool on a wire rack. Store any leftovers in an airtight container for up to 5 days on the counter, or freeze them for up to 2 weeks.

cookie dough date balls

Between leading Baked by Melissa and raising two small kids, I'm always on the go. Sometimes I forget breakfast, sometimes lunch goes late, sometimes I just need a quick pick-me-up between meals. I always have a few of these balls in my bag for my daughters or me when we're running around and need a quick burst of energy. They have nourishing, filling ingredients like almond butter and date caramel, flecks of chocolate chips, and the tempting texture of cookie dough. I keep a stash of these in the freezer, too, for a sweet late-night snack. It's the perfect way to end the day. **MAKES 10 TO 15 BALLS**

1 cup almond flour

¼ cup almond butter, melted

2 tablespoons plus 1 teaspoon maple syrup

2 tablespoons Date Caramel (page 230) or 2 additional tablespoons maple syrup

1 teaspoon vanilla paste or extract

¼ teaspoon fine sea salt

2 tablespoons oat flour

¼ cup dark chocolate chips

½ cup desiccated coconut

1. In a large bowl, combine the almond flour, almond butter, maple syrup, date caramel, vanilla, and salt.

2. Add the oat flour one tablespoon at a time until it reaches a Play-Doh–like consistency. The oat flour acts as an absorption agent and helps solidify the balls as they sit.

3. Add the chocolate chips and mix until combined.

4. Place the coconut in a small bowl or on a plate and roll the dough into 1-inch balls (I like to use a 1-inch ice cream scoop). Roll the dough in the coconut to cover.

5. Store in the fridge in a sealed container for up to 1 week, or freeze for up to 1 month.

tip: If you don't have any oat flour on hand, you can easily make it at home by adding old-fashioned rolled oats to a high-powered blender and pulsing until the oats become a fine powder.

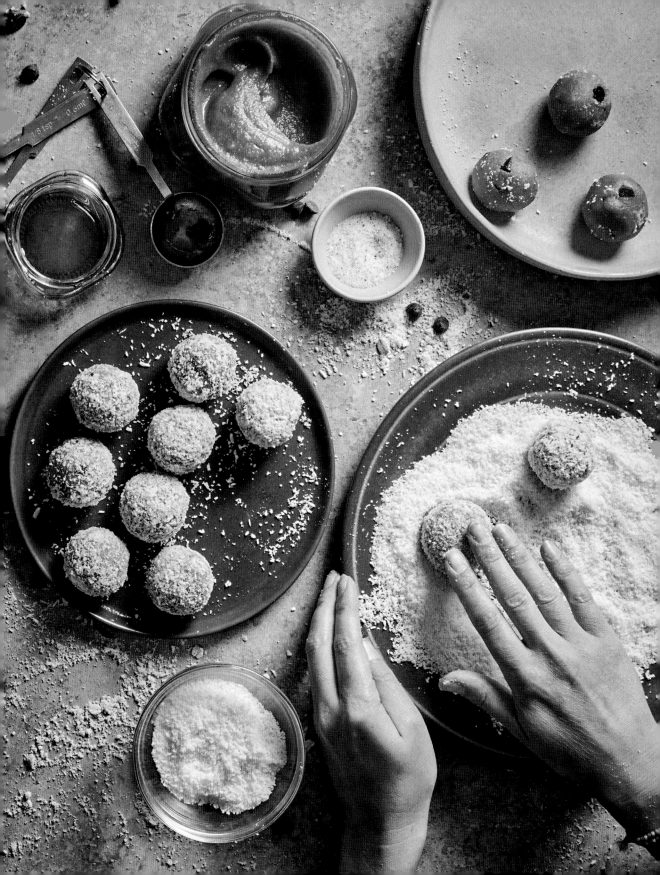

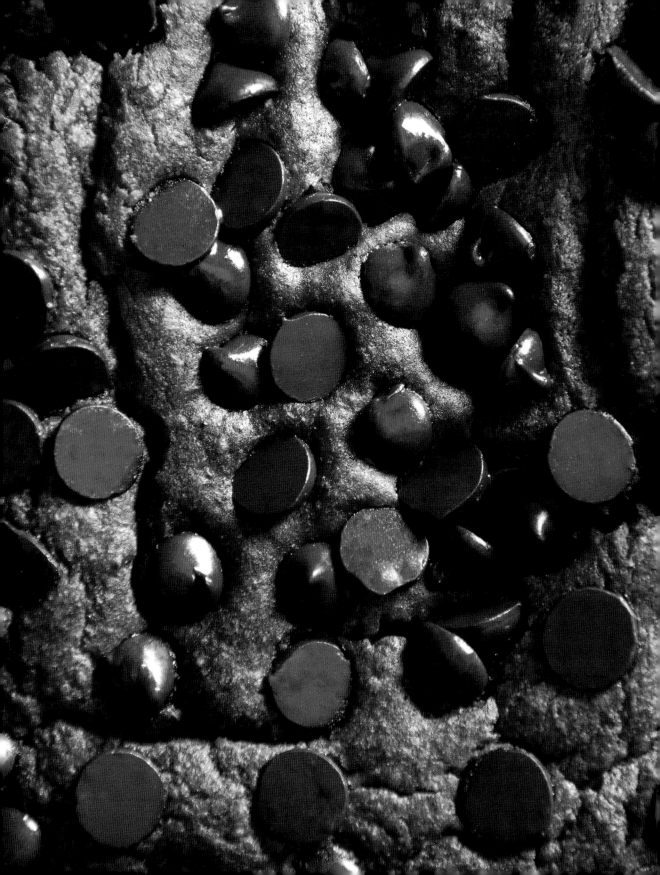

chocolate chip chickpea bread

Just like the Peanut Butter Banana Bread (page 233) and the Double-Chocolate Zucchini Bread (page 238), this loaf cake is a sneaky way to add nutrients to sweets for you and your kids. I make this as a loaf just as often as I make it as muffins. They're easy to pack for breakfast on the go or to freeze to bring on long car trips and flights. I don't know about you, but I always like to have something sweet midflight. **MAKES 1 LOAF**

2 large eggs, at room temperature

3 tablespoons coconut oil, melted

⅓ cup Date Caramel (page 230; you can substitute ⅓ cup maple syrup)

2 teaspoons vanilla paste or extract

3 tablespoons maple syrup

¾ cup full-fat coconut milk

One 15-ounce can chickpeas, drained and rinsed

¼ teaspoon fine sea salt

1½ teaspoons baking soda

1½ teaspoons baking powder

¾ cup oat flour

¾ cup chocolate chips

1. Preheat the oven to 375°F and line the bottom and sides of a 1-pound loaf pan with parchment paper. Leave about 2 inches of parchment paper hanging over the sides to help you pull the bread out later.

2. In a high-powered blender, combine the eggs, coconut oil, date caramel, vanilla paste, maple syrup, coconut milk, chickpeas, salt, baking soda, baking powder, and oat flour until smooth. The batter should be thick.

3. Spread half of the batter across the bottom of the pan and cover with ½ cup of the chocolate chips. Add the remaining batter and top with the remaining ¼ cup chocolate chips.

4. Bake for 50 to 60 minutes, until golden. Remove the loaf from the pan with the parchment paper tabs and cool on a wire rack. Store in an airtight container on the counter for 3 to 5 days, or freeze for up to 2 weeks.

tip: If you want to use this recipe to make muffins instead, just reduce the baking time to 20 to 25 minutes. This will make about 12 muffins.

double-chocolate zucchini bread

Zucchini is one of those magical ingredients that soaks up the flavors around it. So why not make an extra-moist classic chocolate cake with added nutrients? Though typically zucchini breads are made with grated squash, I blended this batter to make everything extra smooth (and, therefore, kid-friendly). It tastes just like chocolate cake, and my kids don't even realize they're eating vegetables in between bites of chocolate chips. **MAKES 1 LOAF**

2 zucchini, ends cut off and chopped into 1-inch-long pieces

½ cup cocoa powder

2 large eggs

1 cup all-purpose flour

½ cup tahina

½ cup maple syrup

3 Medjool dates, pitted

1 teaspoon vanilla extract

1½ teaspoons baking soda

¼ teaspoon fine sea salt

1 cup dark chocolate chips

Flaky sea salt, to garnish

1. Preheat the oven to 350°F and line the bottom and sides of a 1-pound loaf pan with parchment paper. Leave about 2 inches of parchment paper hanging over the sides to help you pull the bread out later.

2. Blend the zucchini, cocoa powder, and eggs in a high-powered blender to combine. Add the flour, tahina, maple syrup, dates, vanilla, baking soda, and fine sea salt and process until smooth.

3. Fold ½ cup of the chocolate chips into the batter.

4. Pour the batter into the loaf pan and cover the top with the remaining ½ cup chocolate chips.

5. Bake for 45 minutes to 1 hour, until a toothpick inserted in the center comes out clean. Sprinkle with flaky sea salt. Remove the loaf from the pan and cool on a wire rack. Store leftovers in an airtight container on the counter for 3 to 5 days, or in the freezer for up to 2 weeks.

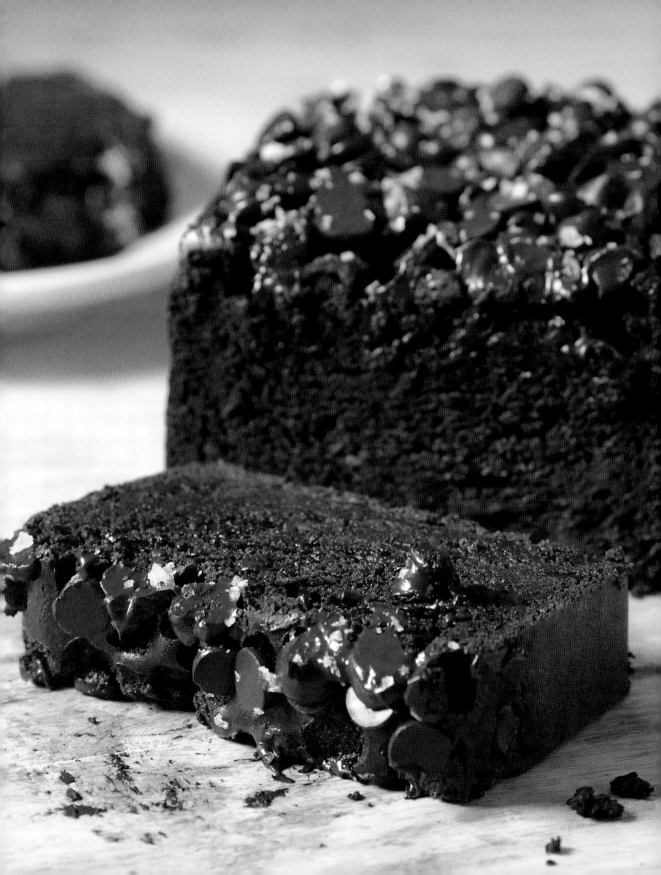

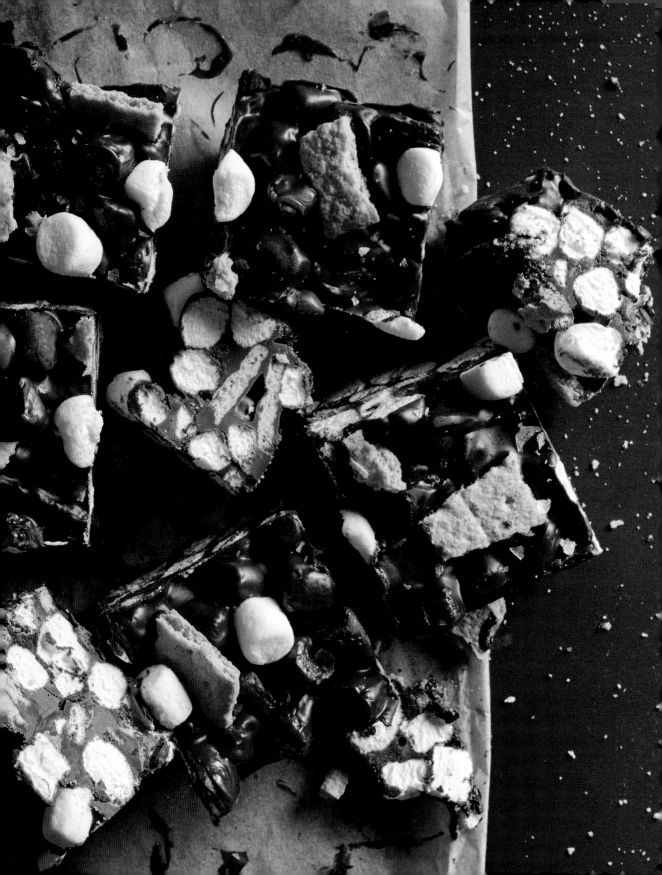

s'mores fudge

It's all in the name—you can never get enough of s'mores. The nostalgic combination of graham crackers, chocolate, and marshmallows reminds me of warm summer nights as a kid and the memories I make with my kids now. If you're having people over or going to a friend's for dinner and forgot about dessert, you can make this in just a few minutes and everyone will love it—I'm sure it'll make them feel like a kid again, too. **SERVES 8 TO 10**

2 cups dark chocolate chips

½ cup creamy peanut butter

9 graham crackers (about 1 sleeve), broken into 1-inch pieces

4 cups mini marshmallows

Flaky sea salt, to garnish

1. Grease an 8 × 8-inch glass baking dish or line with parchment paper.

2. Melt the chocolate chips using a double boiler or by placing a heat-resistant glass bowl over a pot of boiling water, stirring constantly. You can also microwave the chips in 30-second increments until they're fully melted, stirring in between.

3. Once the chocolate is melted, take the bowl off the heat. Stir in the peanut butter.

4. Set aside a small handful each of the graham cracker pieces and marshmallows. Combine the rest in a large bowl.

5. Fold the melted chocolate into the graham crackers and marshmallows until everything is evenly coated.

6. Pour the s'mores mixture into the pan and top with the reserved graham crackers and marshmallows. Freeze for 20 to 30 minutes to cool. Sprinkle with flaky sea salt and cut into individual pieces to serve. Store in an airtight container at room temperature for 3 to 5 days.

s'mores treats

Why would you ever use Rice Krispies for treats when you can use Golden Grahams? (Just kidding. Sort of.) These sweet, delectable treats are like s'mores in a pan, with the cookie butter adding a fudge-like texture. The process of this recipe is very important to get the best results—layering the chocolate chips with the cereal-marshmallow mixture gives you melted chocolate in every bite. You end up with globs of delicious, gooey marshmallows just waiting to be pulled apart and enjoyed.

SERVES 10 TO 12

4 tablespoons (½ stick) unsalted butter, plus more for greasing

½ cup cookie butter (or a nut butter of your choice)

1½ teaspoons vanilla extract

1 teaspoon fine sea salt

5 cups mini marshmallows

One 10.8-ounce box Golden Grahams

1 cup chocolate chips

Flaky sea salt, to garnish

1. Grease an 8 × 8-inch pan with butter or line it with parchment paper.

2. Melt the butter and cookie butter in a large pot over medium heat. Stir in the vanilla and salt. Once melted, add 4½ cups of the marshmallows.

3. Don't let the marshmallows melt fully—they should retain some of their shape. When the marshmallows are three-quarters melted, carefully fold in the Golden Grahams, making sure the cereal is evenly coated with the marshmallow–cookie butter mixture. Remove from the heat.

4. Preheat the oven to broil. Add a layer of the cereal mixture to the bottom of the prepared pan and press down with parchment paper. Top with about ¼ cup chocolate chips and repeat, adding cereal then chocolate, until you reach the top of the pan.

5. Cover the mixture with the remaining ½ cup marshmallows and ¼ cup chocolate chips. Heat under the broiler for 1 to 2 minutes, watching carefully, for a toasty, s'mores-like top. Sprinkle with flaky sea salt and cut into squares to serve. Store any leftovers in an airtight container at room temperature for 3 to 5 days.

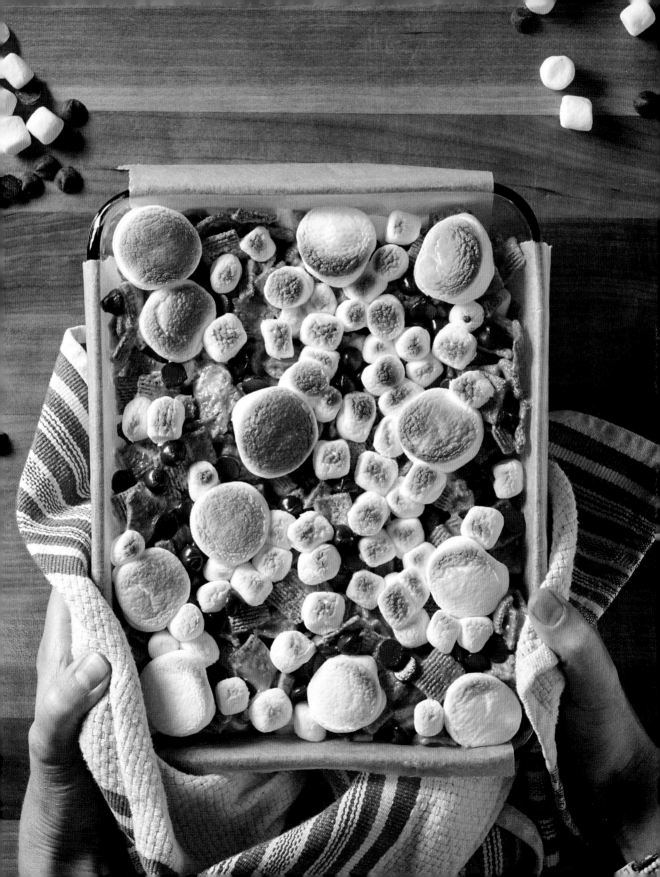

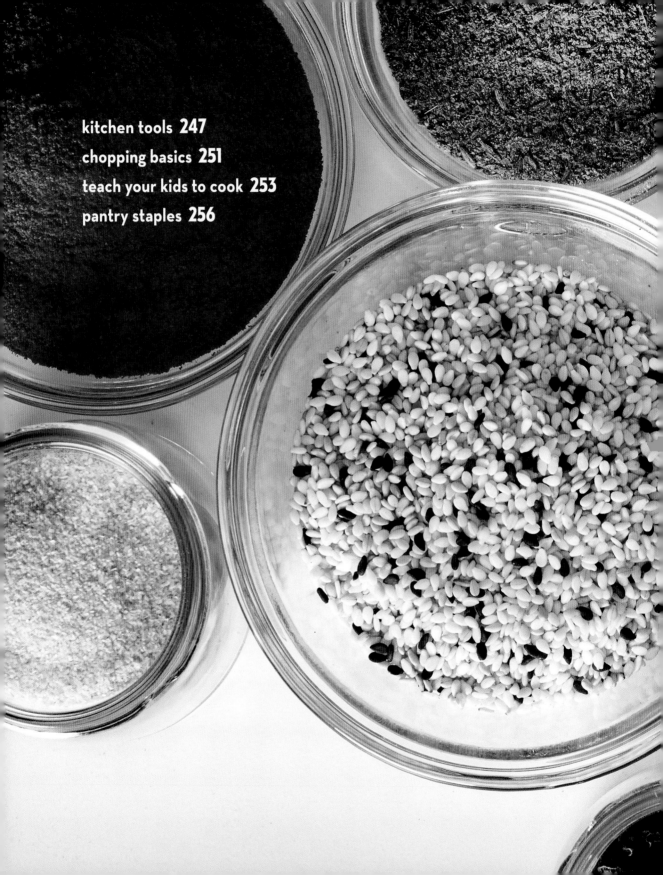

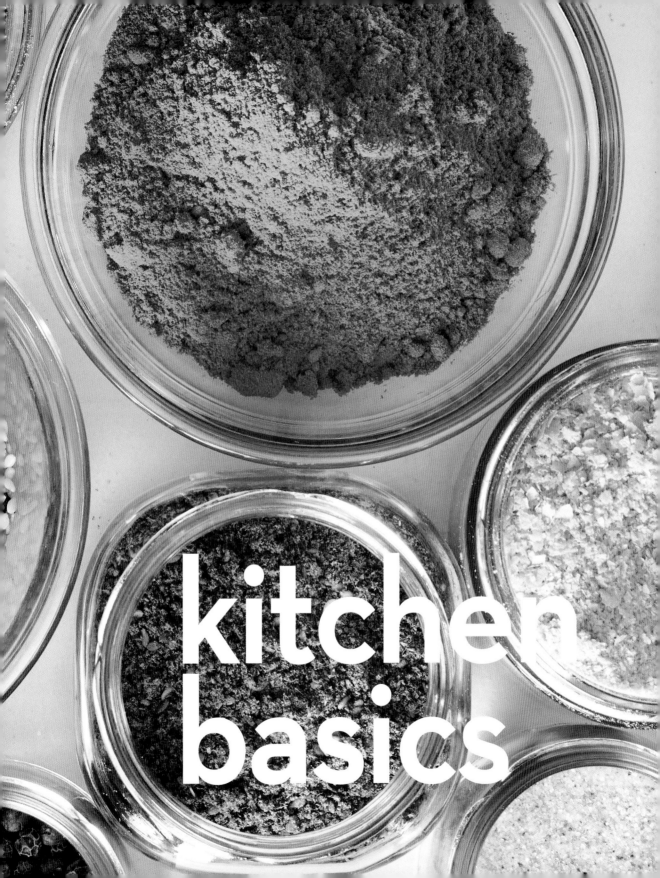

kitchen
basics

kitchen tips i can't live without

- Keep a wet towel next to the cutting board when cutting onions to prevent any tears. The towel absorbs the chemical from the onion that makes you cry before it gets to your eyes.

- To peel garlic, pinch each end of the garlic clove and twist until you hear the crack of the paper releasing from the clove. You should be able to remove all the paper in one piece. It takes practice!

- If you cook with a lot of garlic, save time by storing peeled cloves in an airtight container in the refrigerator. Use within a few days. I find fresh garlic is more flavorful than pre-peeled garlic from the store.

- Invest in a good knife, take care of it, and chop carefully.

- For a quick, easy snack, peel your carrots and store them in an airtight container in the fridge.

- To keep herbs fresh longer, wrap unwashed herbs in a dry paper towel, and store them in a bag in your fridge.

- If you eat a lot of vegetables, a salad spinner is worth the space it takes up.

- Place a damp towel or cloth under a cutting board that simply won't stay in place.

- When making a salad dressing, lemon can be swapped with lime, and almost any vinegar can be substituted with a different variety to get the most of what you have or prefer.

- Always wash sharp knives, pots, and pans by hand to maintain their quality.

- Invest in kitchen equipment you use on a regular basis. A great blender (like a Waring Industrial) will last you a lifetime and make the process smoother and your cooking experience more enjoyable.

- Dress your salad right before serving to keep it crisp.

- Clean as you go—you'll enjoy cooking so much more.

kitchen tools

Every tool in my kitchen has a purpose; ideally, more than one. When kitchen storage is tight, only the best, most useful tools make the cut. I buy tools for function, not beauty, and try to keep them as long as I can by taking care of them and buying quality tools from the start. Many of my go-to utensils are from OXO, like the mandoline, Y peeler, and pastry brush—I love everything I get from them and know the quality is up to par. But with some tools, like the wooden tongs, wooden spoon, and jars, I'm less picky about where they're from—I got the wooden spoon that I use every day for free at an event like ten years ago, and it still does the job well.

- **microplane.** I use garlic in so many recipes, and when I do, I almost always grate it finely with a Microplane, which gives it a sharper, more garlicky flavor. This handy tool is also a must for zesting.

- **wooden tongs.** Whether I'm sautéing vegetables or picking up hot pita, I have these tongs on hand.

- **peeler.** A good peeler takes the task from hassle to joy. You want smooth and effortless strokes to get the job done quickly. Also a plus: It creates gorgeous swirls of produce (like in the Shaved Carrot & Zucchini Salad on page 113).

- **mandoline.** Whenever I want ultra-thin vegetable slivers, especially from cucumbers, radishes, and cabbage, I turn to the mandoline for speed and ease. It also helps slice garlic and onions finely for making homemade powders (like the Garlic and Onion Powders on pages 260 and 261).

- **wooden spoon.** This is a must-have—a good wooden spoon will last forever and prevents scratches on your favorite pots and pans.

- **pastry brush.** I use a silicone pastry brush to cover nooks and crannies of dough with oil and brush on an egg wash for a glossy finish. To improvise, carefully use a spoon. A bonus: Silicone brushes don't shed.

- **small whisk.** I am absolutely obsessed with tiny whisks when making homemade dressings. They fit in almost any container and help emulsify fast.

- **multipurpose knife.** Any good kitchen needs a sharp, reliable knife for chopping, dicing, and slicing. It makes a huge difference in the speed with which I can prep a meal and how well it turns out.

- **tomato knife.** With a delicate serrated edge, a tomato knife gives a cleaner, sharper cut for thin tomato slices and doubles as a tool for crumb-free loaf slices.

- **spatula.** Scrape every last bit of batter or dressing out of the blender, bowl, jar, you name it with a simple spatula.

- **citrus juicer.** I use a simple handheld citrus juicer to get as much lemon juice out of my lemons as possible.

- **bowls of all sizes.** You can never have too many bowls, especially when prepping lots of salads at once. When it comes time to serve, just bring the bowl to the table to enjoy.

- **bench scraper.** Many people use bench scrapers for bread, but they're perfect for quickly scooping up piles of confetti-size veggie chops.

- **scissors.** I promise, when you least expect it, there will always come a time in the kitchen when you wished you had scissors available. I use mine to cut herbs, break down meat, and even to cut up my kids' pizza!

- **jars.** I have a jar collection that's slowly dominating all our pantry space. But these multi-use containers are a must for storing and cooking alike. Nothing excites me more than repurposing a Rao's marinara sauce jar.

- **measuring spoons.** If I'm being honest, I don't measure often. But that doesn't mean you shouldn't, especially if you're new to the kitchen or following a recipe in this book.

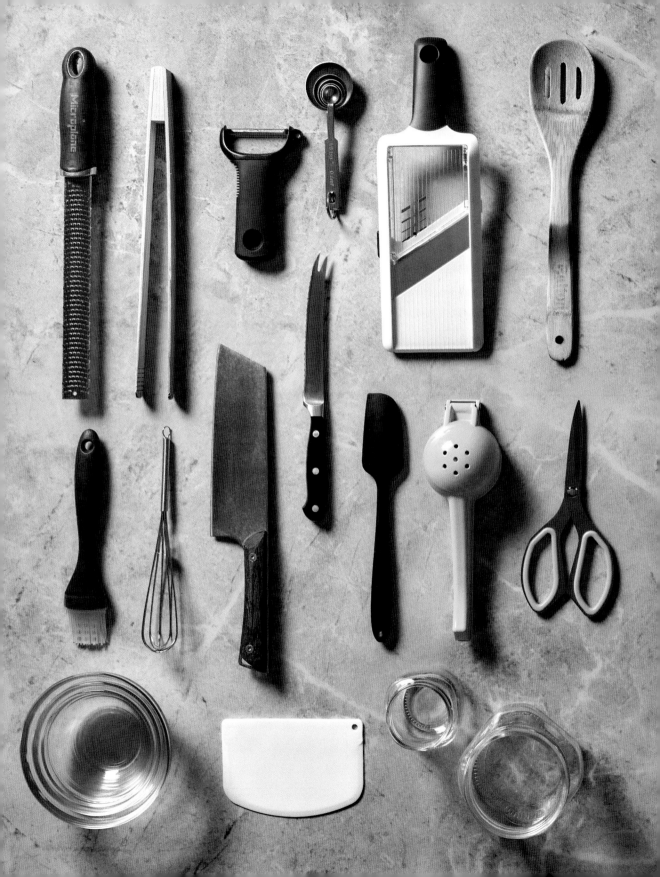

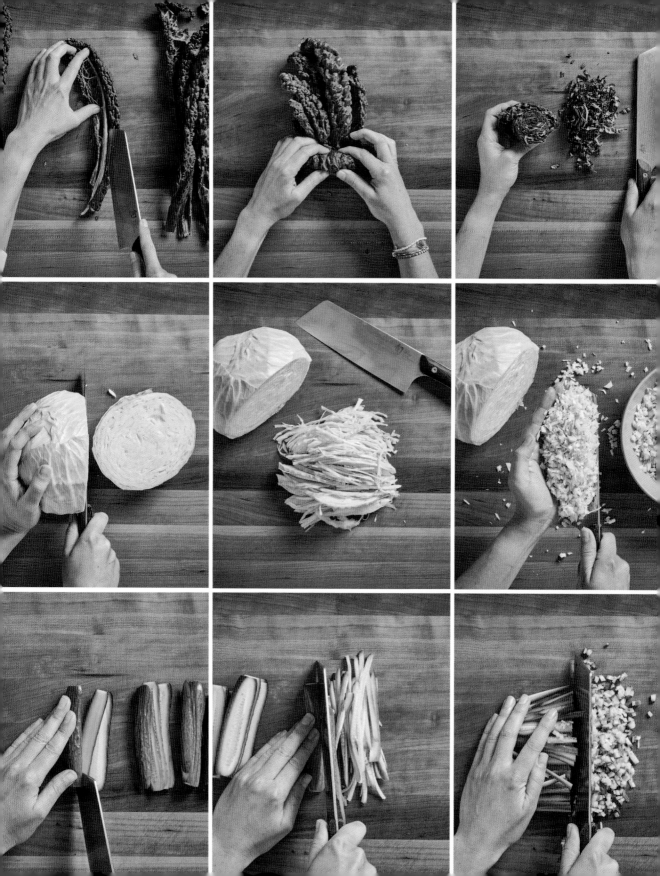

chopping basics

how to chop kale I know many people like to massage kale to make it easier to eat, but I prefer to chop it as small as I can, so it's like confetti. The result is a salad that is packed with kale, but enjoyable with delicious toppings and dressing, too.

1. Lay a leaf of kale flat on a cutting board.

2. Cut out the middle stalk. It's more fibrous and hard to chew.

3. Stack the cut kale leaves together in a pile, as many as you can.

4. Roll the kale up into a spiral.

5. Cut the roll on the short side to create thin ribbons. It should look like grass!

6. For a finer chop, cut the ribbons into smaller pieces.

how to chop cabbage The confetti-size pieces of cabbage are what made the Green Goddess Salad (page 98) such a success. It takes hard-to-eat raw cabbage and turns it into tiny, delightful bits of green. Fair warning: You may end up with pieces of cabbage on the floor. They like to fly away.

1. Cut one-quarter of the cabbage off the head and lay it flat on a cutting board.

2. Starting from one edge, cut it into thin strips. Once you reach the end, turn the entire piece 90 degrees clockwise.

3. Using equally thin strokes, cut the cabbage into small squares the size of confetti.

4. Using the flat side of the knife, scoop the cabbage into a bowl.

how to cut cucumbers I almost always cut my cucumbers into a microchop. They mix well into a salad, are the perfect topping size for a pita, and fit on a chip. Just like with the cabbage, they tend to have a mind of their own, so you might need to sweep afterward. It's worth it.

1. Cut the ends off the cucumbers.

2. Turn the cucumbers lengthwise and cut them into flat strips.

3. Cut the strips into long, thin pieces. Turn them again and cut them into small, confetti-size pieces.

4. Scoop them up with the flat side of the knife and place into a bowl.

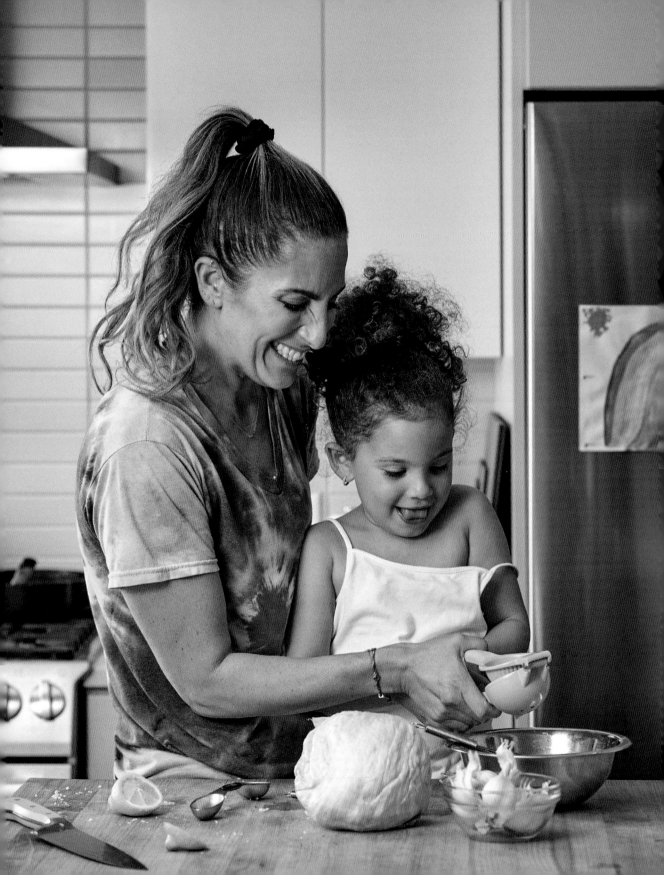

teach your kids to cook

My kids love helping me in the kitchen. They're choosy eaters now, but they handle all kinds of food and feel so accomplished when they help make a delicious meal or snack. Yes, it can get a little (or a lot) messy, but the memories you make now will stay with your kids forever and empower them to get creative in the kitchen.

Here are my tips for including kids in the kitchen (and preserving your sanity).

1. Assign them tasks beforehand. This helps them get excited while staying focused, so they don't make too much of a mess.

2. Premeasure when possible. Measuring ingredients like flour and sugar is much easier with longer arms, so my kids can just pour it into the bowl and feel accomplished.

3. Teach them necessary kitchen skills. Tricks like sliding the spoon across the edge of the baking powder container to create a perfectly even top and learning how to crack eggs are skills you can teach at any age. As my kids got older,

I got them their own knives so they can chop by my side. It's messy sometimes, but it makes them proud.

4. Walk them through the process. Give your kids a heads-up about what's going to happen so they know what to expect and don't get too excited about doing things they can't yet handle.

5. Remember that it won't go as planned. You're inevitably going to have more of a mess to clean up when you invite your kids to cook with you than if you had done it yourself. But the memories are worth it.

6. Try to have fun.

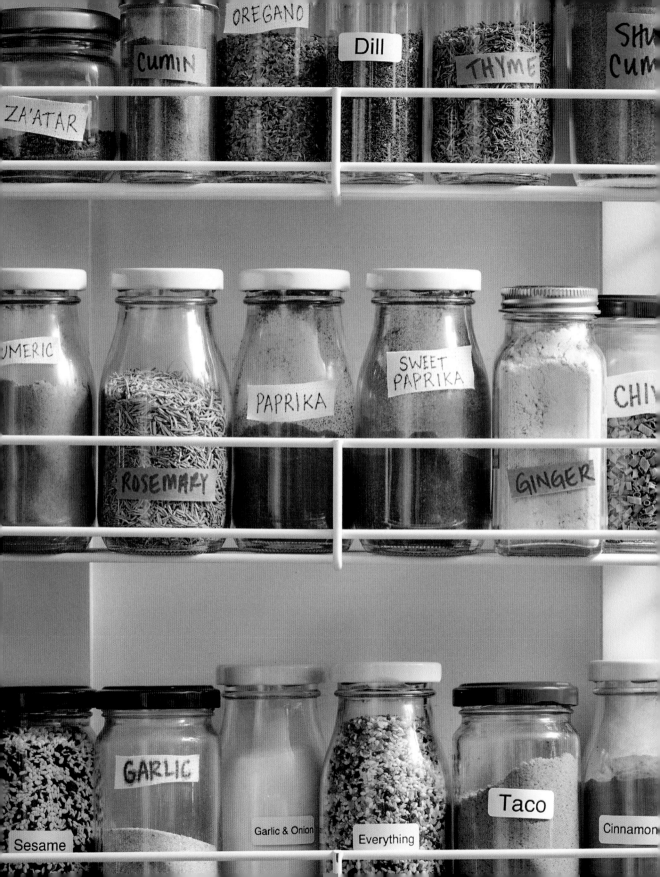

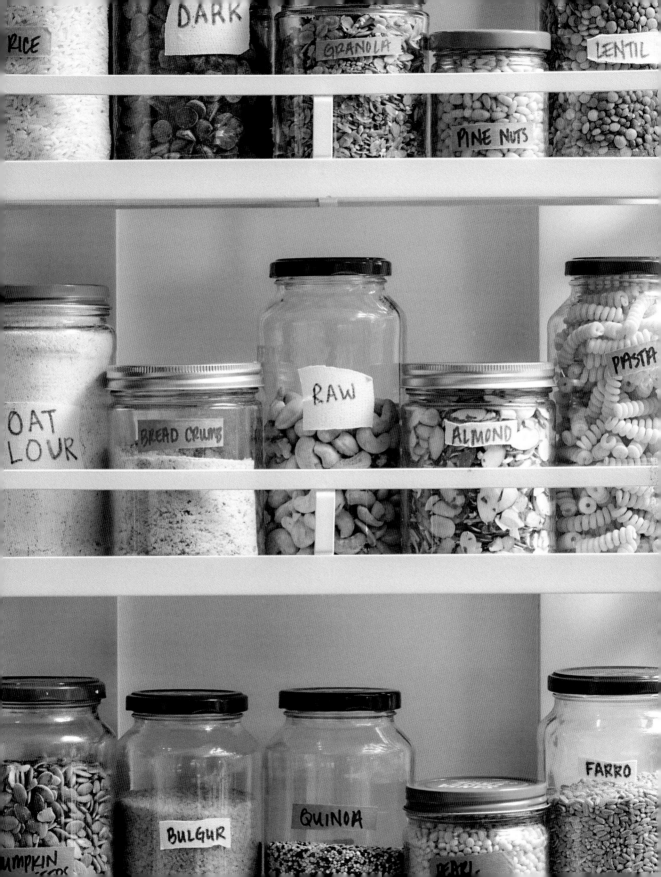

pantry staples

So many of the recipes in this book use pantry staples in fun ways to create meals filled with delicious flavor. With a few basics, you'll have everything you need to whisk up homemade dressing or create a quick dinner. You'll find a few of my most trusted brands below, but ultimately, I want to empower you to discover your favorites and explore the food markets near you, whether they're specialty stores, local farms, a grocery store, or an online shop. All food stores are filled with treasures; you just have to look for them.

refrigerated & produce With these ingredients on hand, creating delicious salads and meals is easy. I buy only organic produce and do most of my shopping on FreshDirect, at Whole Foods, or at the local farmers' market. For the herbs, I've started growing more of them at home so that I can reach for them whenever I need!

- Tahina—We love Lebanon Valley Tahineh Extra, which is sold in huge containers on Amazon and tastes just like what you would get in the Middle East.
- Lemons
- Red Onions
- Yellow Onions
- Shallots
- Scallions
- Cucumbers
- Tomatoes
- Snap Peas
- Carrots
- Fennel
- Olives—Kalamata and Castelvetrano
- Brussels Sprouts
- Chives

- Lettuces—iceberg, romaine, green and red cabbage, little gem, baby butter, spinach, arugula, kale. If you're in the New York City area, I love the greens from Bowery. They're available at many grocery stores and on FreshDirect, are grown without pesticides, and come prewashed. The baby butter lettuce and arugula are especially good.
- Cottage Cheese—Good Culture is the best. The cottage cheese tastes like the delicious creamy inside of a ball of burrata.
- Parsley
- Cilantro
- Dill
- Rosemary
- Thyme
- Dates

spices & seasonings You may have more jars filling your spice cabinet, but these are the tried-and-true staples I reach for most often. If you have a spice shop near you, it never hurts to go in and browse to discover new blends to liven up your spice rack.

- Fine Sea Salt—I use Redmond Real Salt, which has all the nutrients of salt without pollutants.
- Whole Black Peppercorns
- Garlic Powder
- Onion Powder
- Oregano
- Sweet Paprika with Oil
- Sesame Seeds
- Taco Seasoning
- Ground Cumin
- Turmeric
- Za'atar
- Vanilla Paste or Vanilla Extract
- Nutritional Yeast
- Miso Paste

oils & vinegars Make every dressing, marinade, and drizzle imaginable with these staples. Most of these are flexible with what you can find at your local grocery store; I always opt for organic when possible.

- Extra Virgin Olive Oil—I only use Paesanol, a bright-green olive oil from Sicily with a delicious peppery flavor.
- Avocado Oil—I use Chosen Foods, which doesn't have GMOs or additional oils mixed in.
- Toasted Sesame Oil
- White Vinegar
- Rice Vinegar
- Red Wine Vinegar
- Balsamic Vinegar

canned goods When it comes to canned goods, I look for versatility first. Anything that works in more than one way is a keeper. In addition to the other grocery stores I've already named, Trader Joe's has a great canned food selection filled with interesting flavors.

- Tomato Paste
- Tomato Sauce—It's no secret that I love Rao's, and not just because I keep the jars for storage.
- Chickpeas
- Artichoke Hearts
- Hearts of Palm
- Coconut Milk

grains & legumes Create filling meals and add variety to your favorite recipes by swapping out different grains and legumes. Fill your cart with those that excite you wherever you shop—H Mart, Whole Foods, and FreshDirect all have amazing selections.

- Rice
- Rice Noodles
- Farro
- Freekeh
- Quinoa
- Lentils
- Bulgur
- Pasta
- Whole Oats
- Almond Flour

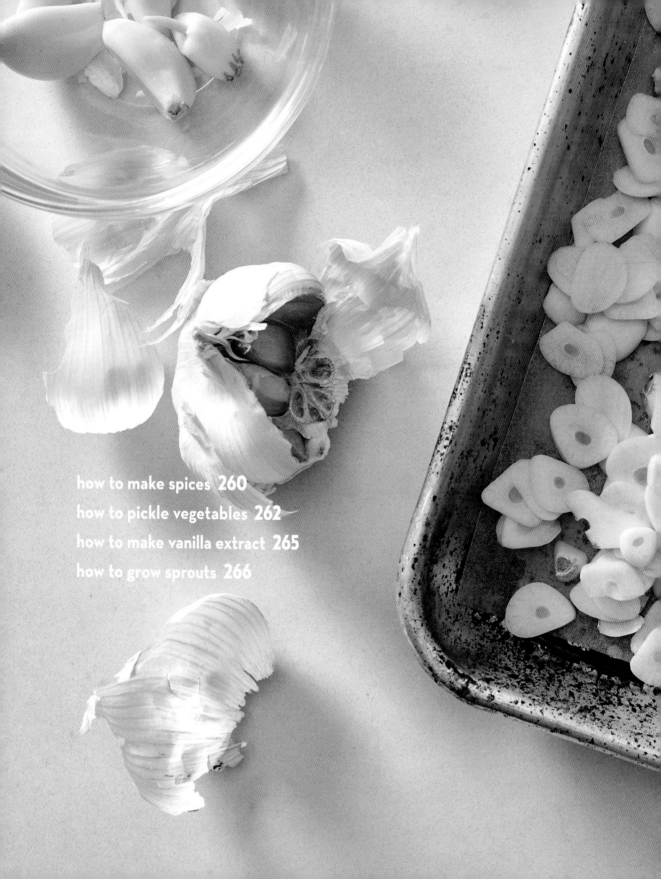

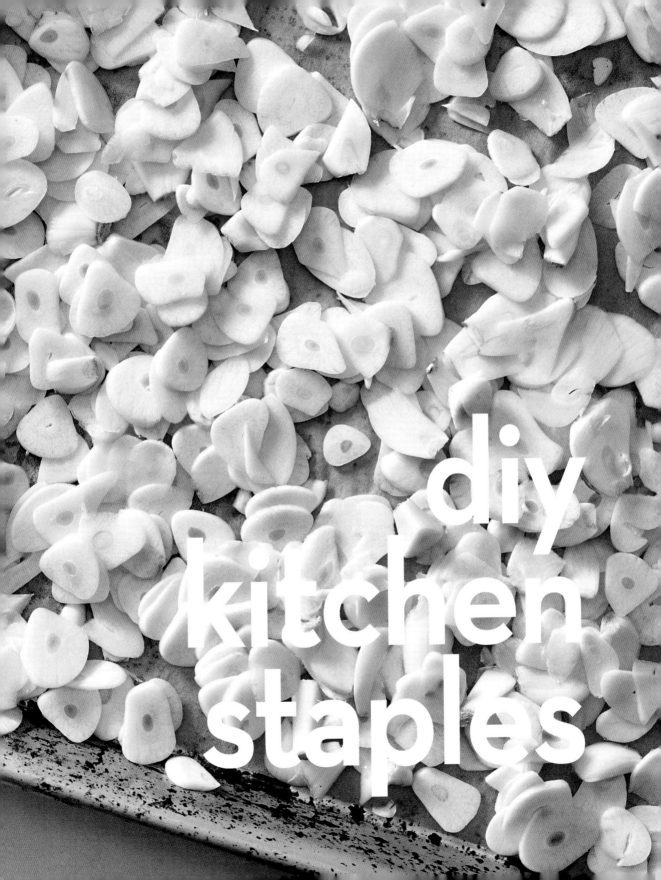

diy
kitchen
staples

how to make spices

One of the biggest revelations I've had in recent years is learning how to make the kitchen staples I use on a regular basis. I love cathartic tasks like peeling garlic, thinly slicing onions, and picking the best-looking herbs from my garden, so it really is a win-win. These spices make great personalized gifts, too—the lucky recipient will always think of you when they use any of what you share. The technique is mostly the same for any herb or spice, but these are my favorites.

garlic powder

Making your own garlic or onion powder is so easy and cost-effective. It can be intimidating because it requires leaving your oven on overnight, but the temperature is so low that it doesn't bother me (of course, please do what's safest for your home!). We have a big wooden bowl in our kitchen to hold all kinds of onions and garlic, and making this homemade spice is how I clean out the ones I've had for a while. You can do it with as many heads of garlic or onions as you like and make them separately or together, but I like to make a big batch to last us a few months. If you love the smell of sautéing garlic and onions, this trick is for you.

6 to 8 heads garlic (or more, depending on how much garlic powder you want)

1. Preheat the oven to 150°F and line a baking sheet with parchment paper.

2. Peel the garlic and slice it into thin slivers using a mandoline (I recommend using a cut-resistant glove to prevent losing any fingertips). The thinner you make the slices, the less time they will take to dehydrate.

3. Arrange the slivers in a thin layer on the baking sheet. (You can use more than one baking sheet if needed.) Place the baking sheet on the middle rack.

4. Cook, stirring the garlic every few hours so that everything dehydrates evenly, for up to 12 hours, or until the garlic feels completely dry. Remove the sheet from the oven. It's very important that everything is fully dried, so I normally leave it out on the counter for 1 to 3 days to make sure. If you're not sure that it's dry, it's not.

5. Add the dried garlic to a blender and pulse until a powder forms. Store in an airtight jar. It stays good for at least 1 year, if you don't finish it sooner.

tip: If I'm making garlic and onion powder combined, I typically aim for a 1:1 ratio.

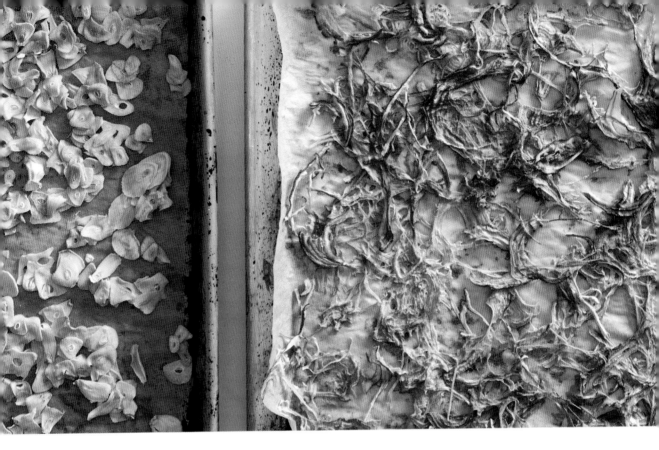

onion powder

4 to 6 large yellow onions, red onions, or shallots, or a combination of all

1. Preheat the oven to 150°F and line a baking sheet with parchment paper.

2. Slice the onion into thin slivers using a mandoline (I recommend using a cut-resistant glove to prevent losing any fingertips). The thinner you make the slices, the less time they will take to dehydrate.

3. Arrange the slivers in a thin layer on the baking sheet—you can use more than one baking sheet if needed. Place the baking sheet on the center rack.

4. Cook, stirring the onions every few hours so that everything dehydrates evenly, for up to 12 hours, or until the onions feel completely dry. Remove the sheet from the oven. It's very important that everything is fully dried, so I normally leave it out on the counter for 1 to 3 days to make sure. If you're not sure that it's dry, it's not.

5. Add the dried onion pieces to a blender and pulse until a powder forms. Store in an airtight jar for up to 1 year.

how to pickle vegetables

We always have at least one kind of pickle, if not more, in our fridge. I love them—they're easy to make and add crunch and tang to anything, whether you're looking for a quick snack or something to add to a pita sandwich. These recipes are the base for delicious pickles, but as you get comfortable with the process, experiment with other herbs and spices you love.

If you aren't sure that pickles are your thing, try the Cucumber & Cottage Cheese Toast (page 51) first. It has a similar flavor profile, but with less bite.

quick-pickled red onions

1 cup white vinegar
1 cup water
1 teaspoon fine sea salt
1 tablespoon maple syrup
1 red onion, thinly sliced

1. Place the vinegar, water, salt, and maple syrup in a saucepan over medium heat. Bring to a rolling boil, then remove from the heat.

2. Add the red onion slices to a 24-ounce jar.

3. Over the sink, carefully pour the vinegar mixture over the onion and cover.

4. Cool to room temperature and seal the jar. Refrigerate the onion for at least 20 minutes or overnight. The pickled onions will keep in the fridge for up to 1 week.

quick-pickled carrots

2 to 3 medium carrots
3 garlic cloves, smashed
1 cup water
1 cup vinegar

1. Slice the carrots into coins and add to a 24-ounce jar with the garlic.

2. In a small saucepan, bring the water and vinegar to a boil over high heat. Remove from the heat and carefully pour the liquid into the jar with the carrots and garlic.

3. Cool to room temperature and seal the jar. Refrigerate the carrots for at least 20 minutes or overnight. The pickled carrots will keep in the fridge for up to 1 week.

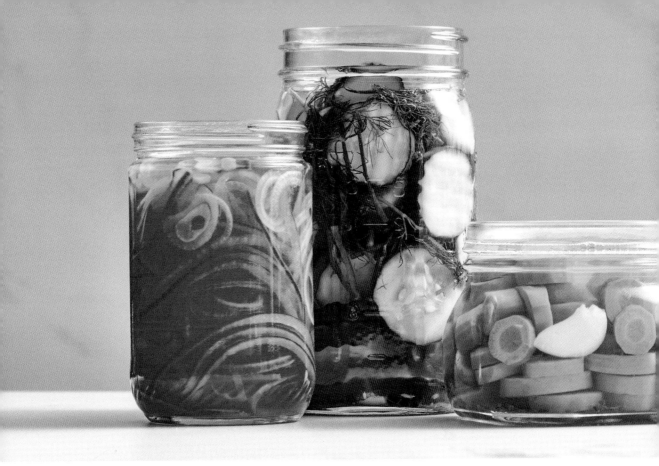

dill pickles

5 garlic cloves
1½ cups water
1½ cups white vinegar
1 tablespoon fine sea salt
1 teaspoon whole black peppercorns
⅓ cup fresh dill, roughly chopped
4 Kirby cucumbers

1. Smash the garlic with the flat edge of a knife to help release the juices. Place the garlic in a small saucepan. Add the water, vinegar, salt, peppercorns, and dill to the saucepan and place over medium heat. Bring to a rolling boil, then remove from the heat.

2. Using a crinkle cutter or knife, cut the cucumbers into ½-inch rounds.

3. Add the cucumber slices to a 32-ounce jar and pour the hot pickling liquid over them until they're completely covered.

4. Allow the cucumbers to come to room temperature, then tightly seal the jar, place in the fridge, and let the cucumbers pickle for at least 24 hours. The pickles will stay good for at least a few weeks, if they last that long.

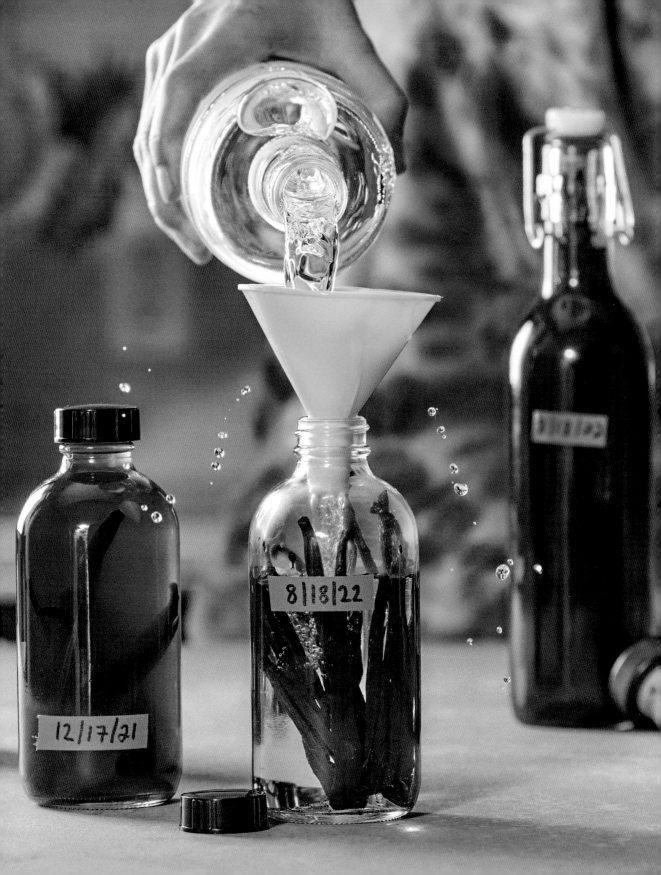

how to make vanilla extract

A few years ago, I started making homemade vanilla extract as gifts for friends. Vanilla beans are expensive, but I promise, this is the gift that keeps on giving. Whenever I use my extracts, I keep the beans in the jar (or bottle, use what you have) and add more vodka to the mix. My vanilla well never runs dry—it's almost as if they're magic beans.

14 vanilla beans

2 cups vodka (I like Ketel One. For my martinis and my vanilla extract.)

1. Slit the vanilla beans lengthwise so the fragrant seeds are exposed. Don't cut them all the way through.

2. Add the beans to a 32-ounce jar and cover with vodka. Tightly seal the jar and store in a cool, dry, dark place like a cabinet or pantry.

3. Let sit for 4 to 6 months, turning the jar occasionally. It should become deep brown in color. Use in baked goods or divide into smaller bottles with a few beans inside to give to friends.

how to grow sprouts

I used to spend so much money buying sprouts at the store. Whenever I make a salad, I'm always looking for new ingredients to add, and sprouts are a winner in so many ways. They're incredibly nutrient dense, versatile, and can add a burst of flavor or volume to a salad. One day I thought: *Sprouts can't be that hard to grow, right?* I *was* right, and now I can't imagine ever buying them again. I use regular mason jars with strainer lids I bought on Amazon and can have a whole crop of fresh sprouts in just a few days. File this under "what can't jars do."

2 tablespoons organic lentils, alfalfa seeds, or broccoli seeds

Filtered water

1. If using lentils, pick them over to remove any debris or stones. Rinse the seeds thoroughly.

2. Add the lentils/seeds to a jar, add filtered water to cover, and soak overnight, or at least 8 to 12 hours.

3. Strain the water in the morning and rinse again, draining the jar well. Store the sprouts jar in a cool, dark place.

4. Do this once in the morning and once at night until your sprouts begin to grow. Basically, you just want to keep the seeds moist so they germinate. For me, it normally takes around 2 to 4 days for seeds to sprout.

5. Use in salads or as a garnish.

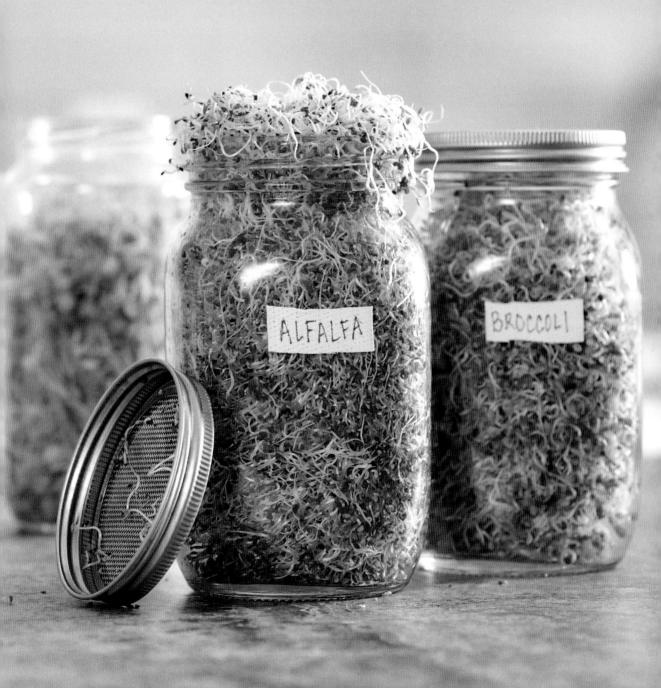

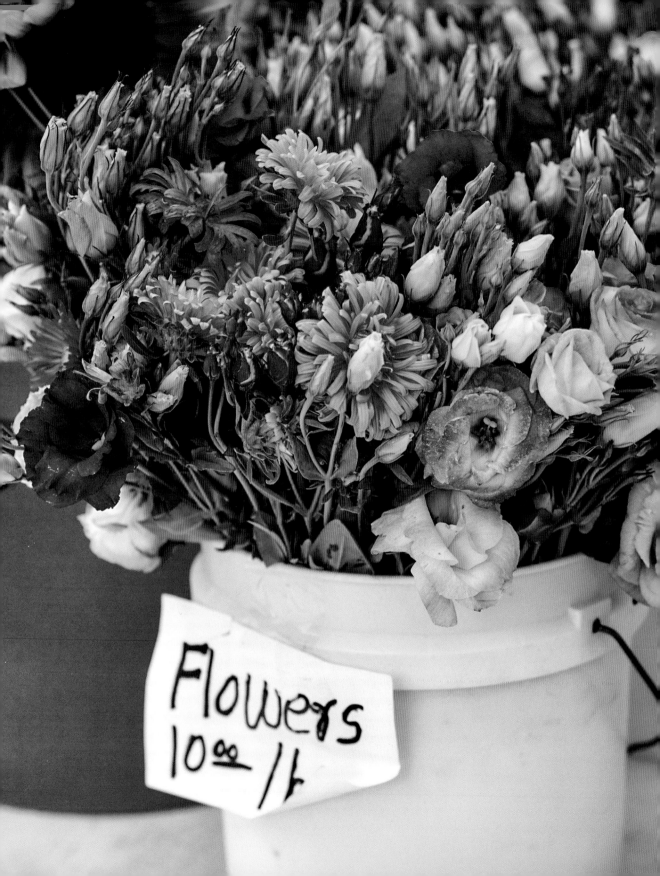

Flowers
10⁰⁰ /lb

acknowledgments

Writing this book was truly a dream come true. It never would have come to be without Adi, who has inspired so much of my cooking over the past fifteen years. This is your book as much as it is mine. Lennie and Scottie, my most delicious girls, you inspire me every day to create the best meals I can (even if you won't eat them . . . yet).

I never would've had the chance to bring these recipes to life if it hadn't been for the incredible Baked by Melissa community, near and far. Thank you for your questions, your inspiration, and for trusting my recipes from the beginning.

To Anne Elder, who joined the Baked by Melissa team in April 2022 as our first-ever content manager and quickly became a friend, confidante, trusted colleague, and unquestionably the person who had to write this book. I cherish the time we have spent working together on this masterpiece and smile with excitement when I think of all the future has in store for us on this magical journey. A special soul and joy to work with, Anne makes me feel privileged to get to work with her every day.

To Megan Reed, who brought this book to life just as much as anyone else. Megan believed in what *Come Hungry* could become even before I did. Her conviction, work ethic, and way with words are unmatched. And it's truly an honor to have her on my team.

To Tsering Dolma, I truly don't know what I would do without you. You take care of me as much as you do my kids, for which I'm eternally grateful. Your positivity and kitchen tricks have made my life infinitely better.

I loved the opportunity to reunite with my creative other half, Ashley Sears, who photographed every recipe in the book (and then some). Her talent for capturing life's most delicious moments is unmatched, and somehow, she does it with ease and patience while keeping the set fun. I'm in awe of your work ethic and professionalism, especially when it comes to caring for your team.

Oak Laokwansathitaya, I so appreciate your support keeping the set energy high and the immense creativity you brought to both the recipe shots and in transforming my rooftop into a floral wonderland. My girls are still asking when they'll see "Green Hair" again. Lauren Damaskinos, every photo in this book is extra crispy thanks to your careful eye; your kindness and positive energy didn't go unnoticed. And Mace Vannoni, your resourcefulness and innovation when it comes to casting the perfect shadow amazes me. A special thanks to Elena Gutierrez, Ian Kornfeld, and Matthew Shrier, too.

Thank you, Lauren Lapenna, Scott Fletcher, and Dominique Lanza, for helping make each and every recipe look its best and teaching me a few food styling tips along the way.

I'm so lucky to have an editorial team who trusted my creativity and let me stretch my legs, including the incomparable Lisa Sharkey, Maddie Pillari, and Iliyah Coles. This book wouldn't be what it is without the extraordinary work of Alison Bloomer, Rachel Berquiest, Emily Fisher, Anna Brower, and the rest of the incredible team at William Morrow.

At Baked by Melissa, so many of our team members helped make this book a success. Meagan Wells, Alyssa Cronin, Ashley Cooper, Elihn Glass, Brittany Attride, Cami Craig, Tessa Widmer, Jennifer Pontrello, and Michaela Keague—I wish I had more space to write about the unique contributions each of you brought to making Come Hungry a success. Thank you for sharing your incredible publicity, marketing, and organizational skills so I can focus on what I do best and create. And to Sam Hahn, who's been with me since the beginning—I hope you love this addition to your cookbook collection. To the Baked by Melissa board of directors, who believed in me and allowed me to grow the brand in so many ways. Words can't describe how much I value your guidance and support.

Endless thanks to all the vendors at the Union Square Greenmarket, who always pulled out the best-looking produce for our photos. Thanks also to PoppyBee Surfaces, Surface Workshop, and Prop Workshop.

Finally, to all the balaboostas—my mom, my grandmothers, my sisters-in-law, and my mother-in-law—and my dad, who pulled up a chair for me at the kitchen counter to teach me how to cook and who showed me that food is love. I couldn't have written this book without you.

universal conversion chart

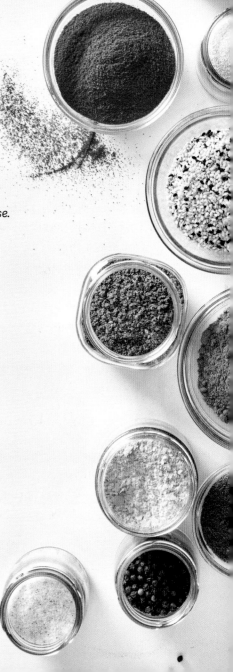

oven temperature equivalents

250°F = 120°C	400°F = 200°C
275°F = 135°C	425°F = 220°C
300°F = 150°C	450°F = 230°C
325°F = 160°C	475°F = 240°C
350°F = 180°C	500°F = 260°C
375°F = 190°C	

measurement equivalents

Measurements should always be level unless directed otherwise.

⅛ teaspoon = 0.5 mL

¼ teaspoon = 1 mL

½ teaspoon = 2 mL

1 teaspoon = 5 mL

1 tablespoon = 3 teaspoons = ½ fluid ounce = 15 mL

2 tablespoons = ⅛ cup = 1 fluid ounce = 30 mL

4 tablespoons = ¼ cup = 2 fluid ounces = 60 mL

5⅓ tablespoons = ⅓ cup = 3 fluid ounces = 80 mL

8 tablespoons = ½ cup = 4 fluid ounces = 120 mL

10⅔ tablespoons = ⅔ cup = 5 fluid ounces = 160 mL

12 tablespoons = ¾ cup = 6 fluid ounces = 180 mL

16 tablespoons = 1 cup = 8 fluid ounces = 240 mL

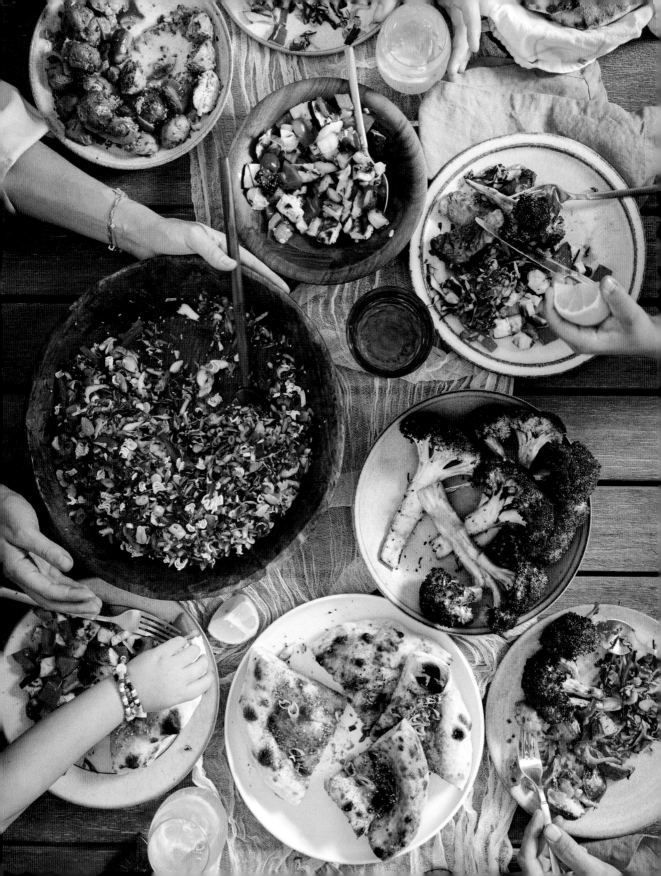

index

NOTE: Page references in *italics* indicate photographs.

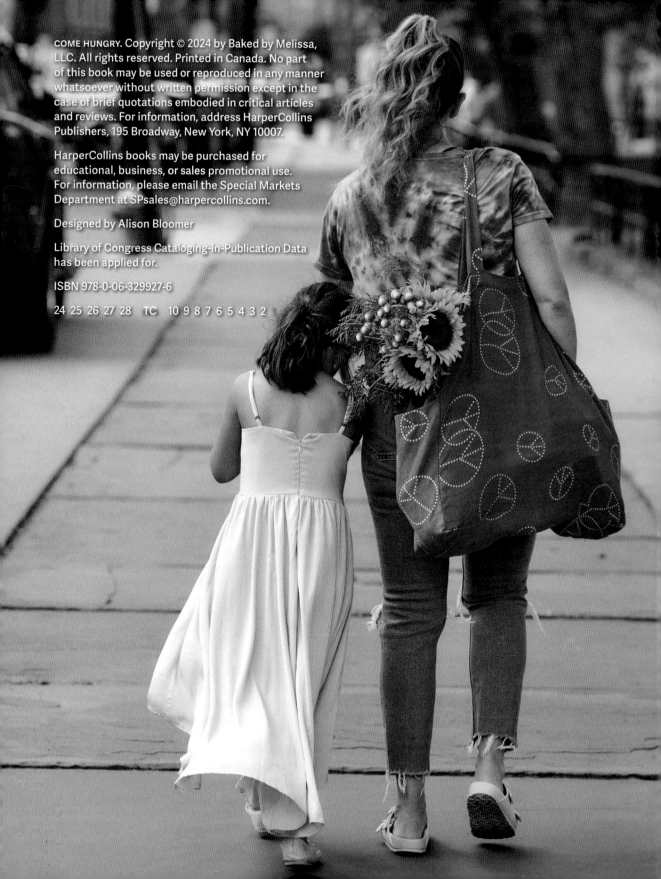

HarperCollins books may be purchased for educational, business, or sales promotional use. For information, please email the Special Markets Department at SPsales@harpercollins.com.

Designed by Alison Bloomer

Library of Congress Cataloging-in-Publication Data has been applied for.

ISBN 978-0-06-329927-6

24 25 26 27 28   TC   10 9 8 7 6 5 4 3 2